Surgical SBAs for Finals with Explanatory Answers

Surgical SBAs for Finals with Explanatory Answers

Thomas Hester
BSc (Hons) MBBS MRCS
Specialist Trainee Year 1
Core Surgical Rotation, Whittington Hospital, London

and

Iain MacGarrow
BSc (Hons) MBBS
Specialist Trainee Year 1
Newham University Hospital, London

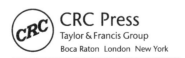

CRC Press
Taylor & Francis Group
Boca Raton London New York

CRC Press is an imprint of the
Taylor & Francis Group, an **informa** business

Radcliffe Publishing Ltd
18 Marcham Road
Abingdon
Oxon OX14 1AA
United Kingdom

www.radcliffe-oxford.com
Electronic catalogue and worldwide online ordering facility.

British Library Cataloguing in Publication Data

A catalogue record for this book is available from the British Library.

ISBN-13: 978 184619 267 8

The paper used for the text pages of this book is FSC certified. FSC (The Forest Stewardship Council) is an international network to promote responsible management of the world's forests.

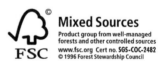

Mixed Sources
Product group from well-managed forests and other controlled sources
www.fsc.org Cert no. SGS-COC-2482
© 1996 Forest Stewardship Council

Typeset by Pindar NZ, Auckland, New Zealand

Contents

Preface

This book is directed at medical students throughout their clinical years, with the questions being a mixture of both clinical and basic science covering the essential topics of surgery. The questions test and reaffirm knowledge with the use of clinical scenarios that should prove to be engaging and make the subject matter more enjoyable and memorable.

Single best answer (SBA) questions are becoming increasingly popular, and can prove a challenge as more than one answer may initially appear to be correct; however, one will be more appropriate than the rest. The book, while detailing the key points in the answers, should hopefully identify areas where further revision is needed.

Thomas Hester
Iain MacGarrow
August 2009

About the authors

Thomas Hester completed a BSc in Orthopaedic Science at UCL and Medicine at St Bartholomew's and the Royal London. He is a regular examiner and instructor on the Royal Society of Medicine revision courses in London. Currently, he is a Core Surgical trainee in London.

Iain MacGarrow graduated in 2006 from St Bartholomew's and the Royal London School of Medicine and Dentistry and is currently an ST1 at Newham University Hospital. He has worked and trained throughout the North East Thames region and is also an Advanced Life Support instructor.

Questions

1 An 11-year-old boy presents to A&E with a five-hour history of vague abdominal pain. On examination he is noted to have a temperature of 38°C, pulse rate of 110 beats per minute, a runny nose and generalised abdominal tenderness that is worse in the right iliac fossa.

What would be the differentiating feature of this condition?
a Raised neutrophils
b Raised lymphocytes
c Raised CRP
d Raised temperature
e Raised white cell count

What bacteria is the most common bacterial cause of this condition?
a *Yersinia enterocolitica*
b *Helicobacter jejuni*
c *Campylobacter jejuni*
d *Salmonella*
e *Shigella*

What radiological investigation would be most appropriate?
a Nil
b Ultrasound
c Computed tomography (appendix protocol)
d MRI
e Abdominal X-ray

The imaging shows some enlarged lymph nodes but is otherwise unremarkable, the patient is currently stable. What is the most appropriate treatment?

a Laparoscopy

b Paracetamol

c Appendicectomy

d Antibiotics

e Watch and wait

2 A 43-year-old lady is referred to A&E by her GP with a 3-day history of 'green' vomit and her stoma is not working. Her past surgical history is significant for a laparotomy 3 years ago for ulcerative colitis complicated by adenocarcinoma of the large bowel that she says was done as an emergency. On examination her temperature is 36.8°C. Pulse is 100 beats per minute regular, BP 120/80. There is midline laparotomy scar, a stoma on the right side with an empty appliance and associated swelling upon lifting head of the bed, the abdomen is soft, non-tender, with no audible bowel sounds.

What is the most likely stoma?
a End ileostomy
b Loop ileostomy
c Urostomy
d End colostomy
e Loop colostomy

What is the most likely cause of her symptoms?
a Recurrence of the tumour
b Strangulated hernia
c Adhesions
d Gastroenteritis
e Pancreatitis

Most appropriate management:
a Laparotomy +/- proceed
b Nasogastric tube placement and intravenous fluids
c Laparoscopy +/- proceed
d Intravenous antibiotics
e CT staging

What is the most likely content of the mass next to the stoma?

a Blood

b Omentum

c Small bowel

d Large bowel

e Bladder

3 A 54-year-old publican presents to A&E with epigastric non-radiating abdominal pain. Past medical history is significant for knee arthritis for which he has been taking voltarol for the past 3 months and has increased his dose in the last 2 weeks. He is overweight but does not smoke. His observations are stable, and the blood results are notable for raised amylase. An admission ECG reveals sinus rhythm, with T wave inversion in leads II, III and aVF.

What is the most likely diagnosis?
a Peptic ulcer disease
b Dyspepsia
c Pancreatitis
d Abdominal aortic aneurysm
e Myocardial infarction

What is the most appropriate management for this patient?
a Triple eradication therapy
b Emergency theatre for operative intervention
c Endoscopy
d Intravenous fluids and nasogastric tube
e Acute coronary syndrome protocol

If bacteria were found to be the principle cause, what would be the characteristic Gram stain?
a Gram –ve bacilli
b Gram +ve diplococci
c Gram +ve rods
d Gram –ve cocci
e Gram –ve rods

What is the pathogenesis of this organism?
a Direct digestion of gastric mucosa by organism
b Produces urea which is directly corrosive to mucosa
c Increase in HCl secretion from antrum
d Increase in HCl secretion from pylorus
e Autoimmune response to bacteria causes ulcer formation

4 A 46-year-old female fast-food employee presents to A&E with a sudden worsening of epigastric pain that radiates to the right upper quadrant and right shoulder tip. On examination she has a large body habitus, is afebrile, with tenderness in the right upper quadrant that arrests inspiration.

What is the most likely diagnosis?

a Hepatitis

b Gallstone disease

c Pancreatitis

d Ascending cholangitis

e Urinary tract infection

What is the most appropriate treatment option?

a Open cholecystectomy

b Laparoscopic cholecystectomy

c Laparoscopic cholecystectomy with on table cholangiogram

d MRCP

e ERCP

She is later found to have a gallstone ileus, what likely finding would support this?

a Raised white cell count

b Deranged liver function tests

c Increased HIDA signal

d A high Glasgow-Imrie score

e Air in the biliary tree on plain X-ray

What is the most likely composition of her gallstones?

a Mixed composition

b Cholesterol

c Bile pigment

d Lecithin

e Calcium oxalate

5 A 73-year-old lady presents to the outpatient department for routine follow up 4 weeks after an abdominoperineal resection, for rectal cancer. She is doing extremely well, and just as she is leaving happens to mention that her left leg has become extremely painful over the past 2 weeks. On examination the left lower leg is erythematous, painful to touch and oedematous, peripheral pulses intact, with no obvious trauma.

What is the most likely diagnosis?

a Cellulitis

b Deep vein thrombosis

c Ruptured Baker's cyst

d Muscle rupture

e Arterial insufficiency

What is the most appropriate initial treatment?

a Intravenous flucloxacillin and intravenous benzylpenicillin

b Subcutaneous enoxoparin 1.5 mg/kg OD

c Warfarin

d None of the above

e a) and b)

Most appropriate investigation?

a Doppler ultrasound

b Intravenous venography

c X-ray AP and lateral

d MRI

e Blood cultures

What is Virchow's triad?

a Lymph node secondary

b Stasis, hypercoagulability, endothelial damage

c Dementia, dermatitis, diarrhoea

d Vertigo, tinnitus, hearing loss

e Free edge of the liver, hepatic duct, cystic duct

6 A 65-year-old smoker, poorly controlled type II diabetic, reluctantly presents to A&E with sudden onset of a painful right leg. He explains that over the past few weeks he has had the pain in his calf when he walks but this settles with rest. Today, however, his leg has become very painful, numb to touch, difficult to move and very cold.

What would be the most useful non-invasive investigation?
a Duplex ultrasound
b ABPI
c Buerger's test
d Angiography
e D-dimers

The surgical registrar on call, upon review, lifts the patient's leg up to 45° and points to venous guttering, then asks the patient to swing their legs over the edge of the bed. What is this test called?
a Rovsing's sign
b Buerger's test
c Trendelenburg's test
d Murphy's test
e Lachman's test

You are asked by the registrar what you think would be your next step?
a Intravenous heparin
b Treatment dose enoxaparin
c Warfarin
d Amputation
e Embolectomy

What is this patient most likely at risk of?
a Myocardial infarction
b Deep vein thrombosis
c Pulmonary embolus
d Varicose veins
e Budd-Chiari syndrome

7 A 62-year-old male, known hypertensive, presents to his GP for routine chronic disease review. On palpation of his abdomen a large pulsatile mass in the midline is found. An abdominal aortic aneurysm was diagnosed.

Which is the most suitable method of imaging for diagnosis?
a CT
b MRI
c Plethysmography
d USS
e Angiography

A 4.5-cm infrarenal aortic aneurysm not involving the iliac arteries is diagnosed. What is the most appropriate course of management?
a Endovascular aortic repair (EVAR)
b Watch and wait
c Emergency repair
d Elective repair

Which of these is NOT involved?
a Medial degenerative disease
b Periadventitial inflammatory and fibrotic response
c *Salmonella*
d Connective tissue disorders
e Hypercoagulability

Which is the most suitable method of imaging for surveillance?
a CT
b MRI
c Plethysmography
d USS
e Angiography

8 A 67-year-old lady with a history of varicose veins and 4 previous pregnancies has a 3-cm sloughy-based ulcer with no associated erythema and is warm to touch. There is pitting oedema to the level of the knee.

What is the most likely location?
a Medial malleolus
b Toe
c Heel
d Foot
e Lateral aspect of foot and ankle

Which of these features is present in arterial disease?
a Intermittent claudication
b Worse at night
c Shiny thin skin
d Atrophic nails
e All the above

Most appropriate management:
a IV antibiotics
b Oral antibiotics
c Compression bandaging
d Surgical embolectomy
e Bypass grafting

The surgical registrar asks you to lie the patient down, elevate the leg, and apply a tourniquet around the upper thigh, then ask the patient to stand up and assess the filling of the superficial venous system. What is this examination called?
a Trendelenburg's test
b Trendelenburg's sign
c Buerger's test
d Buerger's angle
e Lachman's test

9 A 69-year-old female presents to her GP with a 1-week history of being told she looks 'yellow' by her friends. She also complains of itching. On examination there is a mass in the right upper quadrant. She is pain free.

What sign/law is this?
a Trousseau's sign
b Homans' sign
c Courvoisier's law
d Rovsing's sign
e Murphy's sign

What tumour marker would be appropriately measured?
a Ca 19.9
b Ca 125
c Ca 15.3
d AFP
e CEA

If a fine needle biopsy was taken, what would be the most likely finding?
a Adenocarcinoma
b Insulinoma
c Gastrinoma
d Cystadenoma
e Inflammatory changes

The most appropriate surgical management?
a Whipple's procedure
b Roux–en-Y
c Hartmann's procedure
d Lichtenstein repair
e Ramstedt's operation

10 You are asked by your team to see a 55-year-old smoker in pre-admission clinic for repair of an inguinal hernia. He tells you he had three heart attacks in his late 40s and subsequently had an operation but is not sure what he had.

You first note on examination he has a midline incision on his chest. What is the name of this scar?

a Sternotomy

b Thoracotomy

c Laparotomy

d Lanz

e Kocher

What is the likely operation this gentleman has undergone?

a Mitral valve replacement

b Angioplasty

c Coronary artery bypass grafting (CABG)

d Heart transplant

e Pharmacological treatment

You also notice a scar on the medial aspect of his left lower leg. What vein has been harvested?

a Short saphenous

b Long saphenous

c Anterior tibial

d Posterior tibial

e Perforator

On review of his medications, he is currently taking clopidogrel. The mechanism of action is:

a ADP inhibitor

b COX-2 inhibitor

c GIIb/IIIa inhibitor

d Anti Xa

e Nitrovasodilator

11 A 50-year-old male is admitted as an elective right hemicolectomy for a caecal tumour. Seventy-two hours postoperation he develops swinging pyrexia and is tender on palpation of the abdomen.

What type of operation is this?
a Clean
b Clean contaminated
c Contaminated
d Dirty
e Clean dirty

What would be the most likely source of raised temperature day 3 postoperation?
a Basal atelectasis
b Catheter
c Cannula
d Collection
e DVT

The patient develops perfuse watery diarrhoea on day 6 post-operation having received a course of IV cefuroxime and IV metronidazole. What would be the most concerning infection?
a *C. diff* Toxin A
b *C. diff* Toxin B
c *C. diff* 027
d *Campylobacter*
e *E. coli*

How would you treat this patient?
a Intravenous metronidazole
b Intravenous vancomycin
c Oral metronidazole
d Oral vancomycin
e Intravenous fluids

12 A 37-year-old man presents with a painful swelling under the right axilla. On examination he is systemically well, however there are multiple infected foci on the right and evidence of scarring from previous healed foci on the left.

What is the most likely diagnosis?

a   Furuncle

b   Carbuncle

c   Pilonidal abscess

d   Hidradenitis suppurativa

e   Infected sebaceous cyst

Most other likely site?

a   Groin

b   Back

c   Face

d   Breast

e   Natal cleft

Appropriate treatment for this condition is:

a   Watch and wait

b   Oral antibiotics

c   IV antibiotics

d   Incise and drain (I&D)

e   Excision of affected skin

The most worrisome complication if this condition is left untreated is:

a   Recurrence

b   Localised scarring

c   Septicaemia

d   Compression of local structures

e   Self-discharge of pus

13 A 25-year-old cricketer is hit on the side of the head while batting without his helmet on. While mildly concussed he leaves the pitch and is taken home to 'sleep it off'. When his girlfriend arrives home later she is very concerned about how drowsy he is, and phones an ambulance. When they arrive his eyes open to pain, he flexes to pain, and is mumbling incomprehensible sounds.

What is the most likely diagnosis?
a Acute subdural haematoma
b Extradural haematoma
c Subgaleal haematoma
d Subarachnoid haemorrhage
e Overdose

What would be the most appropriate form of imaging?
a CT
b MRI
c PET
d Skull X-ray
e Chest X-ray

Calculate his Glasgow Coma Score (GCS):
a 8
b 9
c 10
d 11
e 12

Most likely vessel involved:
a Middle meningeal
b Internal carotid
c External carotid
d PICA
e Vertebral

14 A 59-year-old lady presents to A&E complaining of a single episode of blindness in her right eye that resolved spontaneously. She
described it using the words 'It was as if someone had shut a cur-
tain in there.'

What is being described?

a   Amaurosis fugax

b   Transient ischaemic attack

c   Stroke

d   Vasovagal attack

e   Cardiac arrhythmia

What would be the next most appropriate line of investigation?

a   Duplex ultrasonography

b   Angiography

c   MRA

d   MRI

e   CT

Most appropriate management for > 70% stenosis would be?

a   Stenting

b   Carotid endarterectomy

c   Bypass graft

d   Balloon angioplasty

e   Conservative treatment

At a later date the patient undergoes surgical management, however postoperatively the patient's tongue is noted to deviate to the
right. What is most likely to have happened?

a   Hypoglossal neuropraxia

b   Glossopharyngeal neuropraxia

c   Haemorrhage

d   Restenosis

e   Partial anterior circulation infarct

15 A 17-year-old boy is blue lighted to A&E with polytrauma following a road traffic accident. You notice instantly that he has two large black rings around his eyes.

What does this finding indicate?

a Basal skull fracture

b Unstable C1-C2 fracture

c Pterion fracture

d Mandibular fracture

e Maxillary fracture

On further examination there is some bruising behind the ears, what sign is this?

a Panda sign

b Grey's sign

c Battle's sign

d Turner's sign

e Cullen's sign

Which airway should be avoided?

a ET

b Laryngeal mask

c NP

d Guedel

e Tracheostomy

Despite aggressive resuscitation he remains hypotensive, you notice his JVP is raised, and on auscultation the heart sounds muffled. What has developed?

a Pericarditis

b Haemothorax

c Dissecting thoracic aneurysm

d Superior vena cava obstruction

e Cardiac tamponade

16 A 30-weeks pregnant lady complains to her GP that she has been getting pain and numbness in her right hand.

How might she further describe this pain?
a   Relieved in cold water
b   Relieved by hanging hand over edge of bed
c   Get better as day progresses
d   Get worse as day progresses
e   Worse after repetition

The GP asks the patient to place her palms together, and extend her wrists, the patient finds this worsens the pain. What is the name of this test?
a   Tinel's
b   Phalen's
c   Chvostek's
d   Trousseau's
e   Uhthoff's

The most likely diagnosis?
a   RSI
b   Osteoarthritis
c   Rheumatoid arthritis
d   Carpal tunnel syndrome
e   Dupuytren's contracture

The treatment for this lady is?
a   Reassure, analgesia and review
b   Elective decompression
c   Emergency decompression
d   Nerve conduction studies
e   MRI

17 A 63-year-old male who underwent oesophagealgastroduodeno-scopy (OGD) unfortunately suffered a perforation. On examination, he is stable but in mild discomfort. Around his neck you can palpate an area that is abnormal, it feels like pressing on cotton wool.

What is this a sign of?
a Lymph node
b Subcutaneous haematoma
c Localised infection
d Local inflammatory reaction
e Surgical emphysema

The most appropriate investigation at this point would be?
a Gastrograffin swallow
b Barium swallow
c Repeat OGD
d Plain abdominal X-ray
e MRI

Which of these conditions may also be associated with oesopha-geal perforation?
a Mallory-Weiss tear
b Boerhaave's syndrome
c Pharyngeal pouch
d Achalasia
e Plummer-Vinson syndrome

The perforation is confirmed in the cervical portion of the oeso-phagus. What is the most appropriate treatment?
a Surgical exploration
b Conservative treatment
c Discharge and follow up in outpatients in 1 week
d Intravenous antibiotics and fluids
e Mediastinoscopy

18 A 56-year-old publican presents to A&E after vomiting blood; he reports this is the first time this has happened. On examination his BP is 130/80, pulse rate 90, respiratory rate 15, and he has a large body habitus. While you are examining him he warns you that his left shoulder has been giving him some trouble and is taking diclofenac for the pain.

What is the most likely diagnosis?

a Oesophageal varices

b Duodenal ulcer

c Mallory-Weiss tear

d Acute gastric erosions

e Gastric ulcer

The most appropriate management is?

a OGD

b Sengstaken-Blakemore tube insertion

c 2 × large bore cannulae and intravenous fluids

d Emergency theatre

e Angiography

Biopsies are taken for CLO testing; what organism does this test for?

a *Helicobacter pylori*

b *Clostridium difficile*

c MRSA

d *Staph. aureus*

e *Strep. pyogenes*

This is negative; what is the most likely cause?

a NSAIDs

b Infection

c Malignancy

d Alcohol

e Idiopathic

19 A 70-year-old female, who has never been to hospital before, reluctantly presents to A&E with a 5-day history of complete constipation. A plain abdominal X-ray shows a massively distended large bowel.

What other imaging should have been performed at this time?

a CXR supine

b CXR erect

c CT chest/abdo/pelvis

d USS abdo

e Barium meal

A sigmoid volvulus is suspected; what treatment should be tried?

a Pass a flatus tube

b Emergency theatre

c Elective theatre

d Barium enema

e Watch and wait

At operation, a sigmoid mass and serosal tears in the caecum; what is the most likely operation to be performed?

a Subtotal colectomy

b Total colectomy

c Hartmann's

d Left hemi

e Right hemi

The small bowel has effluent within its lumen, however it is not distended; what does this tell you?

a There is a metachronous tumour

b The ilio-caecal valve is competent

c Small bowel obstruction

d Coexistent inflammatory bowel disease

e Infective cause for symptoms

20 A 56-year-old male complains of pain and weakness in both legs on standing and on exercise. It is not relieved by rest. He is a non-smoker, with no relevant family history. On examination peripheral pulses are intact.

What is the likely diagnosis?
a   Neurogenic claudication
b   Varicose veins
c   Vascular claudication
d   Peripheral myopathy
e   Osteoarthritis

What would be the most appropriate investigation?
a   MRI
b   CT
c   X-ray
d   USS
e   PET

You note he suffers from arthritis of the hips and knees. On imaging there is some lipping of the vertebral bodies. What is the most likely cause of this finding?
a   Disc prolapse
b   Wedge collapse/fracture
c   Osteophyte formation
d   Ependymoma
e   Secondary deposit

What would be the most appropriate treatment?
a   Conservative
b   Urgent decompression
c   Elective decompression
d   Immobilisation
e   Neoadjuvant therapy

21 A 23-year-old female undergoes an examination under anaes-thesia, however when she is being transferred from the operating table the ODA notices the arm support is incorrectly placed. Postoperatively the patient goes home that evening saying how her hand feels 'funny'. The house officer on call explains that this is likely due to where the drip was sited. Three weeks later in the out-patient department she still complains of some strange sensation.

What is the most likely diagnosis?
a Neuropraxia
b Axonotmesis
c Neurotmesis
d Transection
e Wallerian degeneration

How long will this take to resolve?
a Never
b 1 mm/day
c 6–8 weeks
d 6–8 months
e Partially

What would be the most appropriate mode of imaging?
a CT
b MRI
c X-ray
d Electromyography
e USS

Most appropriate treatment?
a Surgical exploration
b Microsurgery
c Nothing
d Functional splinting and physiotherapy
e Splint alone

22 An elderly gentleman underwent extensive gastric resection and anastomosis without bypass. He reports that he is doing well, his bowels are returning to normal and his appetite is picking up, however he feels noticeably more fatigued since the operation.

What would be a concern?

a Dumping syndrome

b Anaemia: B12 deficiency

c Steatorrhoea

d Anaemia: folate deficiency

e Ulceration

What cells have been removed?

a I cells

b Parietal cells

c Chief cells

d β-cells

e δ-cells

What do these cells produce?

a CCK

b Gastrin

c Intrinsic factor

d HCl

e Folate binding factor

Antibodies to these cells result in?

a Pernicious anaemia

b Folate deficiency

c Microcytic anaemia

d Zollinger-Ellison syndrome

e Myasthenia

23 A 10-year-old male presents to A&E with black loose stool and lethargy.

What is the most likely diagnosis?
a Crohn's disease
b Coeliac disease
c GI bleed
d FeSO$_4$ use
e Recent change in diet

At laparotomy the patient is found to have a mass at 2 feet from the caecum, 2 inches in length that is actively bleeding. The definitive diagnosis is?
a Meckel's diverticulum
b Perforated duodenal ulcer
c Angiodysplasia
d Small bowel lymphoma
e Diverticulum

What is likely to be found on histology?
a Gastric epithelium in particular parietal cells
b Moderately differentiated adenocarcinoma
c Lymphocyte infiltration
d Villous atrophy and crypt hyperplasia
e Normal bowel architecture

What would be the investigation of choice?
a Barium enema
b Technetium scan
c Flexible sigmoidoscopy
d Plain abdominal radiograph
e USS abdomen

24 A 26-year-old Jewish gentleman is referred to clinic by his general practitioner; he complains of several years of relapsing remitting episodes of abdominal pain and bloating, associated with transient increases in stool frequency. He also complains of perianal itching and a mouth ulcer.

What in the social history should be addressed with respect to Crohn's disease?

a Occupational exposure to dust

b ETOH intake

c Smoking

d Weight loss

e Dietary change

Where is Crohn's most likely to be found?

a Mainly anal involvement

b Throughout the colon

c Anywhere from mouth to anus

d Predominately ileal

e Anywhere in small bowel

Which imaging finding is not a feature of Crohn's disease?

a Cobble stone appearance

b Fistula tracts

c Small bowel strictures

d Mesenteric fat stranding

e Rigler's sign

Which option would not be appropriate surgical management?

a Strictureplasty

b Small bowel resection

c Curative colectomy

d Fistulotomy

e Seton placement

25 A 55-year-old woman presents with worsening abdominal pain and distension; she has not had any change in her bowel habit, and she is not clinically jaundiced. She does not complain of any shortness of breath on exertion.

What would be an appropriate tumour marker?
a Ca 125
b Ca 19-9
c Ca 153
d CEA
e AFP

What would be the most appropriate method of imaging?
a USS abdo
b CT abdo/pelvis
c MRI
d CT chest/abdo/pelvis
e Plain abdominal radiograph

Likely diagnosis?
a Diverticular disease
b Ovarian tumour
c Pancreatic tumour
d Sigmoid tumour
e Uterine tumour

What is the cause of distension?
a Malignant transudate
b Malignant exudates
c Low serum albumin
d Infection
e Haemorrhage

26 An elderly patient has been admitted on the previous take with a diagnosis of subacute bowel obstruction. When you examine her you find reduced skin turgor, and dry mucosal membranes with a low urine output (< 0.5 mL/kg/hr).

Where is an important loss of fluid in obstruction?

a 1st spacing

b 2nd spacing

c 3rd spacing

d 4th spacing

e 5th spacing

What is the mostly likely cause of bowel perforation?

a Tumour erosion

b Compression of tissue leading to localised tissue ischaemia

c Mechanical force of bowel distension

d Accumulation of gas in bowel

e Accumulation of toxins in bowel causing local erosion

The most common cause of bowel obstruction is?

a Strangulated hernia

b Carcinoma

c Volvulus

d Adhesions

e Incarcerated hernia

What would be the most appropriate initial management?

a Drip and suck

b Adhesiolysis

c Resection

d Flatus tube insertion

e Encourage oral intake

27 A 70-year-old lady presents with persistent diarrhoea and attacks of facial flushing. A diagnosis of an APUD tumour is made.

Where is the primary tumour most likely to be located?
a Lung
b Sigmoid
c Appendix
d Rectum
e Small bowel

What substance is being secreted?
a Melatonin
b Insulin
c Glucagons
d Serotonin
e Gastrin

What is the secondary tumour location that is responsible for the symptoms?
a Liver
b Brain
c Pancreas
d Bone
e Adrenals

What is the name of this condition?
a Carcinoid syndrome
b Zollinger-Ellison syndrome
c Paraneoplastic syndrome
d Mirizzi's syndrome
e Conn's syndrome

28 An elderly woman presents to A&E with left iliac fossa pain that has been present for the past 3 weeks but has worsened over the last 2 days.

What is the likely diagnosis?
a Diverticular stricture
b Meckel's diverticulum
c Sigmoid tumour
d Diverticulosis
e Diverticulitis

Upon CT scanning you notice that gas is seen in the bladder, what does this indicate?
a Outflow obstruction
b Fistula tract formation
c Sinus formation
d Empty bladder
e Urinary tract infection

What would be the most appropriate operation for this patient?
a Sigmoid colectomy with loop ileostomy
b Hartmann's procedure
c Subtotal colectomy
d Anterior resection
e AP excision

29 A 40-year-old female has a 1-day history of worsening abdominal pain in her left iliac fossa. She is passing flatus and has opened her bowels. Plain abdominal X-ray is unremarkable. What would be the next most appropriate method of imaging?

a USS

b MRI

c CT

d Barium enema

e Barium follow through

Imaging shows partial bowel wall protruding through the femoral canal; what type of hernia is this?

a Richter's

b Spigelian

c Incisional

d Exomphalos

e Gastroschiesis

What is the posterior border of the femoral canal?

a Inguinal ligament

b Psoas muscle

c Pectineal ligament

d Iliacus

e Lacunar ligament

What would be the most appropriate management?

a Emergency theatre

b Drip and suck

c Conservative with light diet

d Elective theatre on planned list

e Needle decompression

30 A 50-year-old obese man complains of epigastric discomfort, and on OGD the OG (oesophageal gastric) junction is noted to be at an abnormal position, though intact, with no other abnormality.

What is the likely diagnosis?
a   Hiatus hernia; sliding
b   Hiatus hernia; rolling
c   Diaphragmatic hernia
d   Congenital hernia
e   *Helicobacter* related gastritis

During examination of the patient you notice that when he is asked to raise his head off the bed there is a large midline mass protruding from the xiphisternum to the umbilicus. What is this likely to be?
a   Congenital diaphragmatic hernia
b   Incisional hernia
c   Traumatic hernia
d   Spigelian hernia
e   Divarification of the rectus

What level does the oesophagus pass through the diaphragm?
a   T8
b   T9
c   T10
d   T11
e   T12

What level is the umbilicus?
a   L1-2
b   L2-3
c   L3-4
d   L4-5
e   L5-6

31 A young patient describes a burning/tearing pain on defecation, and bright red bleeding per rectum. He is otherwise well, though does report a history of migraines. His weight is stable and there is no family history of bowel disease.

What is the most likely diagnosis?
a Fistula in ano
b Fissure in ano
c Haemorrhoids
d Solitary anal ulcer
e Perianal abscess

How would this initially be managed?
a Lifestyle advice, including dietary change
b 2% diltiazem cream topically
c Topical GTN ointment
d Topical Botox injection
e Anal advancement flap

Despite this initial management, he represents to clinic with the same symptoms; what would be the next step?
a Lifestyle advice, including dietary change
b 2% diltiazem cream topically
c Topical GTN ointment
d Topical Botox injection
e Anal advancement flap

32 A known Crohn's disease patient suffers from pain per rectum, has recently been experiencing fevers, and notes some yellow discharge in their underwear.

What is the likely diagnosis?

a Fistula in ano

b Fissure in ano

c Haemorrhoids

d Solitary anal ulcer

e Perianal abscess

What would be the investigation of choice?

a Examination under anaesthesia

b CT

c Endoanal ultrasound

d MRI

e Fistulogram

A 31-year-old male presents to A&E with an extremely tender perianal mass. He is usually constipated. On examination he has a small exquisitely tender mass just outside the anal margin, and does not appear to be protruding from the anal canal.

What is the most likely diagnosis?

a Thrombosed pile

b Anal skin tag

c Anal warts

d Rectal prolapse

e Perianal haematoma

What is the best management for this condition?

a Dietary advice

b Local anaesthetic gel and review in clinic

c Incision and evacuation of haematoma

d Biopsy and review with results

e Delorme's procedure

33 A young man complains of bright red blood on paper and in the pan after passing stool. He also occasionally feels a 'lump come down' when straining.

What is the most likely diagnosis?
a Colonic carcinoma
b Fissure
c Haemorrhoids
d Diverticular disease
e Ulcerative colitis

A 55-year-old lady is seen in the clinic complaining of loose stools and says that she sometimes sees some dark blood mixed in.

What is the most likely diagnosis?
a Colonic carcinoma
b Fissure
c Haemorrhoids
d Diverticular disease
e Ulcerative colitis

A 63-year-old man has a single episode of passing a large volume of blood into the pan that he describes as painless.

What is the most likely diagnosis?
a Colonic carcinoma
b Fissure
c Haemorrhoids
d Diverticular disease
e Ulcerative colitis

A 20-year-old gentleman complains of increased stool frequency that he describes as slimy. What is the most likely diagnosis?

a   Colonic carcinoma

b   Fissure

c   Haemorrhoids

d   Diverticular disease

e   Ulcerative colitis

34 A 54-year-old man presents clinically jaundiced with no discomfort and a palpable mass in the right upper quadrant.

What level is this patient's bilirubin likely to be?

a $> 17\,\mu mol/L$

b $> 35\,\mu mol/L$

c $> 50\,\mu mol/L$

d $> 75\,\mu mol/L$

e $> 95\,\mu mol/L$

In this patient what would be present in the urine?

a Urobilinogen

b Bilirubin

c Neither

d Both

e Bilirubin glucuronide

If you were to ask about this patient's bowel and urinary symptoms, what would he likely report?

a Pale stools, dark urine

b Normal stools, dark urine

c Normal stools, normal urine

d Pale stools, normal urine

What is the likely diagnosis?

a Spherocytosis

b Gilbert's syndrome

c Cirrhosis

d Head of pancreas tumour

e Hepatocellular carcinoma

35 A known alcoholic presents with worsening abdominal distension; what is the likely cause?

a   Heart failure

b   Renal failure

c   Inability to produce albumin

d   Carcinomatosis

e   Chronic peritonitis

Which of the following would be most likely to bleed?

a   Recanalisation of the umbilical vein

b   Collateral between the left gastric vein and the oesophageal vein

c   Retroperitoneal and diaphragmatic anastomosis

d   Inferior and superior rectal vein collateral

e   Splenic hilar varices to retroperitoneum

The patient has difficulty breathing; what is the likely mechanism?

a   Neuropathy

b   Pulmonary oedema

c   Underlying lung disease

d   Splinting of the diaphragm

e   Pickwickian syndrome

What is the most appropriate treatment?

a   Paracentesis

b   Mechanical ventilation

c   IV diuretics

d   Lifestyle change

e   β-2 agonist

36 You are on ITU with your team reviewing a patient with severe pancreatitis.

The registrar asks you what the bruising in the flanks is called?

a Chvostek's sign

b Cullen's sign

c Troisier's sign

d Sister Joseph's sign

e Grey-Turner's sign

What serum marker is not in the Ranson or Glasgow scoring system?

a Urea

b Albumin

c Calcium

d Amylase

e Glucose

If a large mass were palpable within the abdomen, what would be the likely cause?

a Cyst

b Pseudocyst

c Head of pancreas tumour

d Enlarged pancreas

e Distended gallbladder

Another patient is found to present with recurrent peptic ulcers and oesophagitis.

What would be a likely underlying tumour?

a VIPoma

b Adrenocorticotrophin secreting tumour

c Gastrinoma

d Insulinoma

e Prolactinoma

37 A young African female is found to have yellow sclera, and a palpable mass in the left upper quadrant. There is no history of foreign travel, however she says there was some mention of something being wrong with the blood of one of her uncles.

What is the likely diagnosis?

a Malaria

b Schistomiasis

c Lymphoma

d Myelofibrosis

e Sickle cell disease

What is the likely cause of the palpable mass?

a Riedel's lobe

b Spleen

c Carcinoma of the cardia

d Kidney

e Subphrenic abscess

Postoperatively what infection are you most worried about?

a *Staph. aureus*

b *E. coli*

c *Streptococcus pneumoniae*

d *Campylobacter*

e *Staph. epidermidis*

Postoperatively the patient is at increased risk of developing a deep vein thrombosis; why is this?

a Increase in platelets

b Factor V Lieden deficiency

c Protein C deficiency

d Protein S deficiency

e Development of antiphospholipid syndrome

38 Concerning gallstone disease, what is the approximate percentage of mixed stones?

a 75%

b 50%

c 30%

d 25%

e 5%

What percentage is visible on plain abdominal radiograph?

a 5%

b 10%

c 30%

d 70%

e 90%

Bile salts are reabsorbed to re-enter the enterohepatic circulation where?

a Terminal ileum

b Duodenum

c Caecum

d Sigmoid

e Descending colon

What are the fat-soluble vitamins?

a A, D, E and K

b D, E, C and B12

c B12, E, A and D

d K, A, B12 and C

e C, A, D and E

39 A 25-year-old man complains of a dull ache in right scrotum, and is found to have a hard irregular mass on his testicle; you are suspicious of a malignancy.

Which lymph nodes would you expect this to metastasise to?
a Pararectal
b Inguinal
c Para-aortic
d Supraclavicular
e Mediastinal

What would be an associated risk factor?
a Smoking
b Undescended testis
c Inguino scrotal hernia
d Soot exposure
e Trauma

A 15-year-old teenager presents with a sudden onset of acutely painful left testicle. On examination he has a very tender, yet palpable uniformly smooth left testicle and thickened cord.

What is the likely diagnosis?
a Hydrocele
b Epididymo-orchitis
c Testicular torsion
d Torsion of the hydatid cyst of Morgagni
e Inguino scrotal hernia

What is the most appropriate management of this condition?
a USS scrotum
b Plain radiograph to look for bowel gas
c Elective theatre in the morning
d MRI pelvis
e Emergency theatre for exploration

40 A 31-year-old female complains of non-cyclical mastalgia. There is no relevant family history, and on examination there is no obvious mass, only anterior chest wall tenderness.

What is the likely diagnosis?

a Breast abscess

b Tietze's syndrome

c Carcinoma of the breast

d Paget's disease

e Herpes zoster

A 35-year-old female complains of a firm lump in her left breast and says the skin feels thickened. Of note in her past history: she was recently involved in a car crash as a restrained passenger in her boyfriend's car; they both walked away from the crash.

What would be the most likely diagnosis?

a Fat necrosis

b Breast carcinoma

c Fibroadenoma

d Cyst

e Abscess

A 30-year-old woman presents with a firm irregular mass within the right upper quadrant of her breast. There is no nipple discharge or eversion and no lymph nodes are palpable. The lady is very anxious, and her sister has already been diagnosed with breast cancer, aged 42.

What is the likely diagnosis?

a Breast carcinoma

b Cyst

c Fibroadenoma

d Fibroadenosis

e Abscess

What next step should be taken?

a USS
b MRI
c Mammography
d FNA
e Core needle biopsy

41 A patient presents with a large mediastinal mass that is felt to arise from the thymus and is later determined to be malignant.

What is this organ's main function in adults?

a T cell development

b B cell development

c Fat infiltrated redundant organ

d NK cell development

e Stem cell proliferation

The patient is noted to have bilateral ptosis, what is the diagnosis?

a Lambert-Eaton myasthenic syndrome (LEMS)

b Gilbert's disease

c Myasthenia gravis

d Crigler-Najjar syndrome

e Horner's syndrome

If a blood film of a patient with a thymus tumour was analysed, what would most likely be observed?

a Hassall's corpuscles

b Target cells

c Howell-Jolly bodies

d Reed-Steinberg cells

e Heinz bodies

The most appropriate treatment is?

a Pyridostigmine

b Thymectomy

c Thymectomy with radiotherapy

d Donepezil

e Watch and wait

42 With regards to the adrenal gland, which of the following is the single most outer layer?

a Zona glomerulosa

b Zona reticularis

c Zona fasciculata

d Cortex

e Medulla

A patient, after extensive investigation for hypertension, is found to have Conn's syndrome; what is in excess?

a Aldosterone

b Epinephrine

c Hydrocortisone

d ACTH

e 17-α hydroxyprogesterone

What electrolyte abnormality may be found?

a Decreased potassium

b Increased potassium

c Decreased sodium

d Increased calcium

e Decreased calcium

What would be the most appropriate treatment for a patient with this condition?

a Open adrenalectomy

b Laparoscopic adrenalectomy

c Spironolactone

d Frusemide

e Lifestyle changes

43 A 40-year-old female presents to her GP with a large painless swelling in her neck. Her thyroid appears enlarged and has several palpable lumps. Upon checking her thyroid function, she is euthyroid.

What would be the most likely diagnosis?

a Multinodular goitre

b Colloid goitre

c Endemic goitre

d Hyperplasia

e Papillary carcinoma

What would be the most appropriate treatment for this condition?

a Radioactive iodine 131

b Propylthiouracil

c Carbimazole

d Subtotal thyroidectomy

e Total thyroidectomy

Which of the following is the most common thyroid cancer?

a Papillary carcinoma

b Follicular adenoma

c Anaplastic carcinoma

d Medullary carcinoma

e Thyroid lymphoma

What other condition is associated with medullary carcinoma of the thyroid?

a Phaeochromocytoma

b Small cell lung carcinoma

c Lymphoma

d Malignant myeloma

e Renal oncocytoma

44 Which of the following does parathyroid hormone regulate?

a Calcium

b Potassium

c Calcium and phosphate

d Sodium

e Magnesium

Peribuccal tingling is a sign indicative of what in the post-thyroidectomy patient?

a Damage to the facial nerve intra-operatively

b Low potassium

c Low calcium

d Damage to the recurrent laryngeal nerve

e Vascular insufficiency

The registrar asks you to inflate a BP cuff on the patient's arm, which you do and note that there is carpopedal spasm; what sign is this?

a Trousseau's sign

b Chvostek's sign

c Lhermitte's sign

d Uhtoff's sign

e Rovsing's sign

45 After a urethral catheterisation, you notice an hour later that the patient's glans has become grossly swollen.

What is this diagnosis?
a Phimosis
b Paraphimosis
c Non-retractable prepuce
d Erection
e Balanitis

The initial treatment for his condition is?
a Pressure to glans with local anaesthetic block
b Urgent circumcision
c Dorsal slit
d Venous decongestion with syringe
e Arterial decongestion with syringe

A diabetic patient presents with balanitis; what organism do you consider before prescribing appropriate treatment?
a *E. Coli*
b *Staph. epidermidis*
c *Streptococcus*
d *Staph. aureus*
e *Candida*

If a carcinoma were suspected, which lymph nodes would most likely be affected?
a Pararectal
b Inguinal
c Para-aortic
d Supraclavicular
e Mediastinal

46 You are called to the ward to review a patient who has lost consciousness after what the nurse describes as a heavy fall, broken only by his head after tripping on his walking frame. She tells you he is on warfarin for atrial fibrillation, and she is worried.

At what point should intubation be considered?
a GCS < 12
b GCS < 10
c GCS < 8
d GCS < 6
e GCS < 4

You are concerned about this patient's airway. What immediate airway intervention would you administer?
a Laryngeal mask + O_2
b Nasogastric tube + O_2
c Nasopharyngeal airway + O_2
d Endotracheal tube + O_2
e Guedel airway + O_2

What do you think the likely diagnosis would be?
a Subdural haematoma
b Extradural haematoma
c Subgaleal haematoma
d Subarachnoid haemorrhage
e Overdose

His INR is found to be 8; what would you ideally like to give him?
a Vitamin K oral
b Vitamin K IM
c Fresh frozen plasma
d Platelets
e Prothrombin complex

47 A young man presents to A&E with severe right sided flank pain, and microscopic haematuria. A diagnosis of ureteric colic is made.

What would be the most sensitive form of imaging?
a Plain abdominal radiograph
b CT KUB
c IVU
d USS
e MAG3 scan

What proportion of ureteric stones are seen on plain KUB films?
a 5%
b 10%
c 30%
d 70%
e 90%

Most appropriate analgesia:
a Pethidine
b Morphine
c Paracetamol
d Tramadol
e Codeine

Primary treatment of this condition is?
a Extracorporeal shock wave lithotripsy
b Ureteroscopy – electrohydraulic lithotripsy
c Open ureterolithotomy
d Laparoscopic ureterolithotomy
e Ureteroscopy with use of Darmia basket

What type of stones does a proteus infection predispose to?

a Oxalate

b Phosphate

c Uric acid

d Cystine

e Urate stones

48 A 60-year-old smoker who used to make Wellington boots presents to the urology clinic after a GP referral for haematuria. He is pain free with only the occasional clot seen. He is on warfarin, his most recent INR being 2.5 yesterday.

Where is the likely location of the bleeding?
a Kidney
b Ureter
c Bladder
d Prostate
e Urethra

What would be the most appropriate investigation?
a IVU
b CT
c USS
d Flexible cystoscopy
e Urine MCS

The appearance is of a malignant tumour; what is it most likely to be?
a Transitional cell papilloma
b Transitional cell carcinoma
c Squamous carcinoma
d Adenocarcinoma
e Sarcoma

What would be the most appropriate next step?
a TURBT
b TURP
c Intravesicle chemo
d Intravesicle BCG
e Cystectomy

49 A 65-year-old male has difficulty passing urine; his wife, who accompanies him, says he is getting up more than normal in the night to go to the toilet.

What percentage of males over 70 have benign hyperplasia of the prostate?

a 10%

b 30%

c 50%

d 70%

e 90%

After investigation to rule out a suspicious cause, he is started on tamsulosin; what is the mechanism of action?

a Selective α-1 adrenergic antagonist

b Non-selective α-1 adrenergic antagonist

c 5-α reductase inhibitor

d Prevents the conversion of testosterone to dihydrotestosterone

e Prevents the conversion of dihydrotestosterone to testosterone

The patient continues to have symptoms despite this treatment, and undergoes a TURP. Postoperatively he initially does well, but his wife reports that he does not seem himself and is becoming increasingly confused; he also complains of nausea. His observations are stable and bladder irrigation fluid is flowing very well. Bloods are sent to the lab and reveal hyponatraemia. What is the likely diagnosis?

a Internal haemorrhage

b TURP syndrome

c Urinary infection

d Bladder neck stenosis

e Worsening of existing cerebral degeneration

50 A lady in need of a kidney transplant is due to have one donated by her twin sister.

What is this type of graft known as?

a Allograft

b Isograft

c Xenograft

d Autograft

e Heterograft

What term best describes the location of this graft?

a Orthotopic

b Heterotopic

c Anatomical

d Regional

e Isotopic

Which of the following is not an exclusion criterion for a potential donor?

a Potential transmission of infection

b Malignancy

c Impaired donor organ function

d Low grade primary brain tumour

e Current substance abuse

What are the 1- and 5-year quoted survival rates for patients who undergo renal transplant?

a 90% and 60%

b 95% and 65%

c 80% and 70%

d 75% and 50%

e 95% and 80%

51 Which of the following is associated with varicose veins?

a Atrophie blanche

b Acanthosis nigrans

c Lipodermatosclerosis

d Necrobiosis lipoidica diabeticorum

e Pretibial myxoedema

What should be excluded before operating on varicose veins?

a Arterial insufficiency

b Deep venous insufficiency

c Superficial insufficiency

d Perforator insufficiency

e Varicose skin changes

What is the most common site of incompetence?

a Saphenofemoral junction

b Femoraliliac incompetence

c Profunda femoris incompetence

d Popliteal incompetence

e None of the above

What would be sought before using compression stockings for treatment of a varicose vein related venous ulcer?

a Angiography

b ABPI

c USS duplex

d Plain radiograph

e Tourniquet test

52 An elderly gentleman presents with diffuse muscle wasting throughout his right leg, which he says has been present since childhood. Upon asking him to stand you notice that he has bowing of the knees.

What is this deformity called?

a   Hallux valgus

b   Genu recurvatum

c   Genu valgus

d   Genu varus

e   Pes plannus

Upon standing on his right leg his pelvis dips to the left. What muscle group is likely to be affected?

a   Left adductors

b   Left abductors

c   Right adductors

d   Right abductors

e   Left quadriceps

What is the likely diagnosis?

a   Polio

b   Guillain-Barré syndrome

c   Charcot-Marie-Tooth disease

d   Friedrich's ataxia

e   Muscular dystrophy

What part of the neurological system is destroyed by the poliovirus?

a   Neuromuscular junction

b   Anterior horn cells

c   Dorsal root ganglion

d   Sympathetic chain

53 You are asked to see a 73-year-old lady with a large ulcer over the medial malleolus of her left foot. There is a healthy base, with granulation tissue present. There are superficial dilated veins over the medial aspect of the leg.

What is the likely diagnosis?
a Venous ulcer
b Arterial ulcer
c Marjolin's ulcer
d Curling's ulcer
e Cushing's ulcer

What would be the most appropriate treatment?
a Antibiotics
b Graduated compression stockings
c Varicose vein striping
d Debridement
e Split skin graft

Before treating, what investigation must be performed?
a Wound swab
b Duplex ultrasound
c Biopsy
d X-ray
e Angiography

The ulcer becomes chronic. On inspection the appearance has changed and now has heaped edges. What is the diagnosis?
a Venous ulcer
b Arterial ulcer
c Marjolin's ulcer
d Curling's ulcer
e Cushing's ulcer

54 A diabetic 55-year-old gentleman presents to A&E with a dark black toe. On examination, there is no exudate present and the toe is not painful.

What is the diagnosis?

a Dry gangrene

b Wet gangrene

c Acute digital ischaemia

d Traumatic injury

e Severe cellulitis

What would be the most appropriate treatment?

a Elective amputation

b Emergency amputation

c Auto-amputation

d Emergency angioplasty

e Elective angioplasty

His pedal pulses are present; what is the likely reason for this?

a The ulcer is neuropathic

b Microvascular disease

c Large vessel disease

d Poor technique and you are actually palpating your own digital pulses

What would be the likely ABPI in this gentleman?

a > 1

b 0.8

c 0.5

d < 0.3

e A compressible pulse at 50 mmHg

55 Having been asked to examine a gentleman's abdomen you find a pulsatile, expansile mass in the midline above the umbilicus. The patient is otherwise well, with no precipitating event, and his VDRL test is negative.

What is the likely diagnosis?

a Iliac aneurysm

b Abdominal aneurysm

c Thoracic aneurysm

d Transmitted pulse

e Mesenteric aneurysm

What is the most appropriate initial imaging modality?

a Ultrasound

b CT

c MRI

d Aortogram

e X-ray

The mass is found to be 5.6 cm in diameter, 1.4 cm infra renal, and does not extend to involve the iliac arteries. What is the best treatment?

a Elective open aneurysm repair

b Emergency open aneurysm repair

c Elective EVAR

d Emergency EVAR

e Watch and wait

The most likely cause of this gentleman's aneurysm is:

a Traumatic

b Atherosclerotic disease

c Syphilitic degeneration

d Connective tissue disease

e Idiopathic disease

56 You see a young 25-year-old male as part of your OSCE examination. He has a 5 cm by 5 cm swelling over his forearm, with a transverse surgical incision over the surface. On examination the mass is pulsatile and expansile with a palpable thrill.

What is the likely diagnosis?

a Brachiocephalic fistula

b Radiocephalic fistula

c Pseudoaneurysm

d True aneurysm

Upon auscultation of the mass you would hear:

a Pansystolic murmur

b Machinery murmur

c Ejection systolic murmur

d Early diastolic murmur

e Late diastolic murmur

The patient later develops a painless swollen hand with no evidence of erythema; the radial pulses are palpable. What is the likely cause?

a Steal phenomena

b Thrombosis

c Infective arthropathy

d Autoimmune reaction

e Fistula breakdown

Another patient with the same mass presents with worsening pain on using his right hand; there are weak pulses.

What is the likely cause?

a Steal phenomena

b Thrombosis

c Infective arthropathy

d Autoimmune reaction

e Fistula breakdown

57 A 65-year-old man presents with a painless, pulsatile swelling in the back of his right knee. What is the most likely diagnosis?

a Baker's cyst

b Semimembranous bursa

c Popliteal vein aneurysm

d Popliteal artery aneurysm

e Knee capsule cyst

What are the associated complications of this condition?

a Arterial thrombosis

b Compression of popliteal vein

c Rupture

d Compression of tibial nerve

e All of the above

What is the most appropriate form of imaging?

a Ultrasound scan

b Angiography

c CT angiography

d MR angiography

e Plain radiograph

The mass identified is 1.8 cm in diameter and is asymptomatic. The most appropriate treatment of this condition is:

a Vein bypass

b Dacron graft

c PTFE graft

d Embolise

e Leave and observe

58 A young man presents with multiple subcutaneous soft masses that are not attached to the overlying skin or to the underlying tissue. They are painful if pressure is applied to them. What is the likely diagnosis?

a Lipoma

b Dercum's disease

c Lipomatosis

d Neurofibroma

e Leiomyoma

Treatment of the lesions is best carried out by:

a Excision

b Biopsy

c Observe

d Routine bloods

e Ultrasound scan

Multiple benign papilloma associated with an underlying malignancy is known as:

a Leser-Trelat syndrome

b Sister Joseph's nodule

c Trousseau's sign

d Dercum's disease

e Von Recklinghausen's syndrome

Port-wine staining on a patient's leg, together with superficial dilated veins is:

a Parkes-Weber syndrome

b Osler-Weber-Rendu syndrome

c Klippel-Trenaunay syndrome

d Sturge-Weber syndrome

59 An elderly gentleman presents to his GP with a painless mass on his upper arm that becomes more prominent upon actively flexing his elbow. There is no history of any trauma. What is the most likely diagnosis?

a Ruptured proximal biceps tendon

b Ruptured distal biceps tendon

c Ruptured proximal triceps tendon

d Ruptured distal triceps tendon

e Ruptured brachialis muscle

What is the most appropriate treatment for this condition?

a Emergency open repair

b Elective open repair

c Watch and wait

d Functional bracing

e Synthetic cast in 45° of flexion

A 45-year-old school teacher experienced a tearing sensation in her right calf while playing squash and has subsequently noticed that she is scuffing the right toe of her shoes.

What test is likely to be positive on examination?

a Simmond's test

b Trendelenburg's test

c Gerber-Ganz test

d Lachman's test

e McMurray's test

What is the most appropriate treatment for this condition?

a Emergency open repair

b Urgent open repair

c Watch and wait

d Functional bracing

e Synthetic cast in 45° of flexion

60 A fair-skinned lady presents with a non-tender mass on her left arm. It is purple/black in nature, with an irregular border and a friable flat surface.

This is likely to be:
a Acral lentiginous melanoma
b Superficial spreading melanoma
c Nodular melanoma
d Lentigo maligna melanoma
e Pigmented naevus

A Nigerian lady presents to your practice; she has noticed a black lesion on the sole of her foot. She has never noticed it before.

What is this likely to be?
a Acral lentiginous melanoma
b Superficial spreading melanoma
c Nodular melanoma
d Lentigo maligna melanoma
e Pigmented naevus

What does a Hutchinson's lentigo run the risk of developing into?
a Acral lentiginous melanoma
b Superficial spreading melanoma
c Nodular melanoma
d Lentigo maligna melanoma
e Pigmented naevus

A 40-year-old lady presents to you because she has recently read a Sunday newspaper article about skin cancer. She has had a lesion on her left shoulder all her life, which has not changed colour or bled and has been 0.5 cm in diameter for as long as she can remember.

What is the most likely diagnosis?
a Acral lentiginous melanoma
b Superficial spreading melanoma
c Nodular melanoma
d Lentigo maligna melanoma
e Pigmented naevus

61 A 23-year-old male attends to the GP because his hands have become unbearably painful in cold weather. He is a builder and smokes 20 cigarettes a day. There is no family history of any illness. On examination there are palpable pulses, with good capillary refill.

What is the likely diagnosis?

a CREST syndrome

b Raynaud's disease

c Raynaud's phenomenon

d Scleroderma

e Acrocyanosis

What is the most appropriate management?

a Lifestyle changes

b Nifedipine

c Digital amputation

d Cervical sympathectomy

e IV prostacyclin

What are the associated skin changes to this particular condition?

a Calcinosis

b White, blue, crimson change in skin colour upon warming of cold hands

c Skin tethering

d Multiple telangiectasia

e Multiple lipomas

Upon further questioning you discover that this patient also reports difficulty swallowing and has some other interesting skin changes. What is the likely diagnosis?

a CREST syndrome

b Acrocyanosis

c Erythrocyanosis frigida

d Bazin's disease

62 A patient seen in clinic complains of profuse sweating from the hands, axilla and feet.

The likely diagnosis is:

a Hyperhidrosis

b Hidradenitis suppurativa

c Hyperhidrosis erythematous traumatica

d Frey's syndrome

e Syringomyelia

A young man presents to A&E with an axillary abscess. There are multiple old scars from previous drainage, and the axilla is likened to a watering can by the registrar.

What is the diagnosis?

a Hyperhidrosis

b Hidradenitis suppurativa

c Hyperhidrosis erythematous traumatica

d Frey's syndrome

e Syringomyelia

He is systemically well, and there is minimal associated erythema. The most appropriate course of action is to:

a Commence IV antibiotics

b Incision and drainage

c Complete axillary clearance

d Cervical sympathectomy

e Painting with aluminium hexachloride

After the initial presentation with appropriate management, what would be the most definitive treatment?

a Commence IV antibiotics

b Incision and drainage

c Complete axillary clearance

d Cervical sympathectomy

e Painting with aluminium hexachloride

63 An elderly gentleman has been referred to the general surgical clinic for a mass that is apparent on coughing in the upper midline of the anterior abdominal wall. On examination you notice a large scar in the midline. This is likely to be:

a Epigastric hernia

b Diverification of the rectus

c Incisional hernia

d Lipoma

e Sister Joseph's nodule

The gentleman is otherwise well with no other comorbidity, other than a BMI of 32. He opened his bowels earlier that day. He finds the mass sometimes becomes larger and uncomfortable and would like something done about it. What would be the most appropriate course of action?

a Emergency open repair

b Emergency laparoscopic repair

c Elective open repair

d Elective laparoscopic repair

e Yearly follow up

64 A 47-year-old male patient presents with a non-tender swelling in his left scrotum. It is about 2.5 cm in diameter, well-defined, smooth, firm and fluctuant. It transluminates and lies separate to the testicle and behind the cord which is separate.

What is the likely diagnosis?
a Maldescended testis
b Varicocele
c Hydrocele
d Epididymal cyst
e Testicular cancer

You examine a young man, who complains of an enlarged right scrotum. It is soft mass, which can be felt separate from the testicle. The cord structures can be felt through the swellings, which feel like a 'bag of worms'.

What is the likely diagnosis?
a Maldescended testis
b Varicocele
c Hydrocele
d Epididymal cyst
e Testicular cancer

A 27-year-old man presents with a non-tender mass in his scrotum, the testicle cannot be felt separately, however the epididymis can. The mass is firm and does not transluminate. What diagnosis must be excluded?
a Maldescended testis
b Varicocele
c Hydrocele
d Epididymal cyst
e Testicular cancer

An elderly gentleman presents with a large scrotum. On examination you find that it is restricted to the right; you cannot palpate the testicle separately. The mass transluminates.

What is the likely diagnosis?

a Maldescended testis

b Varicocele

c Hydrocele

d Epididymal cyst

e Testicular cancer

65 You are asked on the ward round to comment on a gentleman's abdomen. You see a midline scar and a pink stoma flat to the surface of the abdomen with brown stool in the appliance. The patient had an AP excision.

What is the likely diagnosis?

a Ileostomy

b Colostomy

c Urostomy

d Ileal conduit

e Jejunostomy

Upon lifting his head you see a mass around the stoma that was not previously present. What is this?

a Incisional hernia

b Inguinal hernia

c Prolapse

d Parastomal hernia

e Hernia retraction

The patient reports that sometimes the mass stays and the stoma does not work, but normally settles down. He has noticed it for the last year. He is otherwise fit and well. What would be the treatment of this?

a Emergency repair

b Elective repair

c Watch and wait

d Resiting of the stoma

e Reversal of the stoma

66 An elderly gentleman is seen in clinic with longstanding groin pain. On examination his left leg lies in external rotation, with a degree of fixed flexion. His gait is antalgic but he can weight bear. He is otherwise well, has never experienced any trauma, is not on steroids and has only suffered from this condition over the last 3 years.

What type of shortening would be present?

a   True shortening

b   Apparent shortening

c   Tibial shortening

d   Fibula shortening

e   Femoral shortening

What test would you use to determine the fixed flexion?

a   Thomas's test

b   Trendelenburg's test

c   Lachman's test

d   McMurray's test

e   Buerger's test

What is the likely diagnosis?

a   Osteoarthritis

b   Rheumatoid arthritis

c   Paget's disease

d   Perthes' disease

e   Avascular necrosis

67 What test would be used to determine if the deep venous system of the leg was patent?

a Perthes' test

b Trendelenburg's test

c Tourniquet test

d Buerger's test

e ABPIs

How would you determine the level of valve incompetence?

a Perthes' test

b Trendelenburg's test

c Tourniquet test

d Buerger's test

e ABPIs

Which test determines saphenofemoral incompetence?

a Perthes' test

b Trendelenburg's test

c Tourniquet test

d Buerger's test

e ABPIs

Your registrar asks you to demonstrate if a patient develops reactive hyperaemia due to peripheral vascular disease.

What test would show this?

a Perthes' test

b Trendelenburg's test

c Tourniquet test

d Buerger's test

e ABPIs

68 On examination of a patient's knee you find a thickened capsule. What disease process is this indicative of?

a Osteoarthritis

b Rheumatoid arthritis

c Polio

d Osteochondritis dissecans

e Ehlers-Danlos syndrome

In which condition may genu recurvatum be most commonly seen?

a Osteoarthritis

b Rheumatoid arthritis

c Polio

d Osteochondritis dissecans

e Ehlers-Danlos syndrome

A 13-year-old girl is brought to the GP's by her mother; on examination, she has pain over the tibial tuberosity.

What is the diagnosis?

a Chondromalacia patellae

b Osgood-Schlatter

c Osteochondritis dissecans

d Tibial exostosis

e Housemaid's knee

What would be the most appropriate treatment?

a Arthroscopy

b Simple analgesia

c Osteotomy

d Tendon release

e Aspiration

69 An elderly lady is seen on the ward round. The consultant asks you what the bony lesions are on the distal phalanges.

They are:
a Rheumatoid nodules
b Heberden's nodes
c Bouchard's nodes
d Osler's nodes
e Virchow's node

Another elderly lady has ulnar deviation of the metacarpal phalangeals.

What else might you see at the elbow?
a Rheumatoid nodules
b Heberden's nodes
c Bouchard's nodes
d Osler's nodes
e Virchow's node

Which joint is hyperextended in a Boutonniere deformity?
a Proximal interphalangeal joint
b Metacarpophalangeal joint
c Distal interphalangeal joint
d Radial deviation
e Ulnar deviation

Which joint is hyperextended in Swan neck deformity?
a Proximal interphalangeal joint
b Metacarpophalangeal joint
c Distal interphalangeal joint
d Radial deviation
e Ulnar deviation

70 A 40-year-old male presents with a fixed flexion deformity of his ring and little finger.

Which gene mutation is linked to this condition?
a ZF9
b BRCA 1
c BRCA 2
d HLA B27

To assess the functional deficit which test will you ask the patient to perform?
a Houston's test
b Froment's test
c Finklestein's test
d Tinel's test
e Phalen's test

While this is being performed, what other incidental finding might you make which would be associated with this condition?
a Rheumatoid nodules
b Heberden's nodes
c Bouchard's nodes
d Osler's nodes
e Garrod's pads

71 You are asked to examine a patient; when your registrar asks the patient to place his hands against the wall with his arms outstretched, you notice a prominent right scapula.

Which nerve is likely to have been affected?

a Radial nerve

b Median nerve

c Ulnar nerve

d Long thoracic nerve

e Musculocutaneous nerve

Another patient in clinic is asked to place his hand on the table and point his thumb directly up to the ceiling, which he is unable to do.

Which nerve is affected?

a Radial nerve

b Median nerve

c Ulnar nerve

d Long thoracic nerve

e Musculocutaneous nerve

Which nerve is tested for by Froment's test?

a Radial nerve

b Median nerve

c Ulnar nerve

d Long thoracic nerve

e Musculocutaneous nerve

Upon sensory examination of a patient's left hand, you find loss of fine touch over the first web space.

Which nerve is affected?

a Radial nerve

b Median nerve

c Ulnar nerve

d Long thoracic nerve

e Musculocutaneous nerve

72 A 26-year-old man presents to the Emergency Department complaining of pain in his right hand after falling over the previous Saturday night.

Which of the following assesses ulnar nerve function in the hand?

a Active wrist flexion and extension

b Active finger abduction and normal sensation over ring and little finger

c Active finger abduction and normal sensation over index and middle finger

d Normal sensation in the anatomical snuffbox

e Ability to actively oppose thumb and little finger

On examination, the patient has normal ulnar, radial and median nerve function and has a normal capillary refill time in all fingertips. He is tender over the little finger metacarpal in the right hand, with accompanying swelling. There is no open wound. What imaging should you request?

a AP and oblique right hand views

b AP and oblique little finger views

c Scaphoid views

d AP and lateral right wrist

e CT right hand

Radiographs reveal a fracture of the neck of the little finger metacarpal with palmar angulation of less than 15°. What is the appropriate immediate management of this injury?

a Futura splint

b Neighbour splint of little and ring fingers

c Full hand POP cast

d K-wiring +/- ORIF

e Ulnar gutter splint

What is the likely mechanism causing this type of fracture?

a Fall onto dorsiflexed hand
b Fall onto palmarflexed hand
c Punching hard object
d Crush injury to hand
e Hand struck with sharp object

73 A six-and-a-half-year-old child presents to the Emergency Department having fallen while playing on a climbing frame; her parents say that she fell onto her outstretched hand. On examination, the child is distressed and will not let anyone touch her left arm. She is holding her elbow in extension and complains of pain throughout the arm. The ED has requested radiographs.

What is the usual order of ossification in the paediatric elbow?

a Olecranon, radial head, medial epicondyle, lateral epicondyle, trochlea, capitellum

b Capitellum, radial head, medial epicondyle, trochlea, olecranon, lateral epicondyle

c Medial epicondyle, lateral epicondyle, trochlea, olecranon, capitellum, radial head

AP and lateral radiographs of the left elbow reveal a supracondylar fracture. What eponymous grading system is used to categorise these fractures?

a Weber

b Rolando

c Garden

d Gartland

e Catterall

Which of the options below is the most important to assess in this child?

a Neurovascular status distal to the injury

b Symptoms and signs of head injury

c Bony injury in the wrist and hand

d Range of movement at elbow

e Check for any open wounds

The radiographs reveal complete posterolateral displacement of the distal part of the humerus. What is the appropriate definitive management?

a MUA and K-wiring

b ORIF

c Collar and cuff

d Broad arm sling

e Above-elbow backslab

74 You are the house officer on call at the weekend and are asked to review a 60-year-old lady who is currently being managed conservatively for a diverticular abscess. You find an alert but uncomfortable lady, who looks hot and sweaty. Her urine output is around 30 mL/hr (her weight is 70 kg), BP is 106/63, HR 103 and temperature 37.6°.

After you have taken a brief history and examined her what should you do next?

a Fluid challenge, repeat bloods

b Reassure patient and nursing staff

c Chest X-ray, abdominal X-ray

d Continue with current management but review in an hour

You are called away and eventually return to review the patient 4 hours later. She says she feels better; her observations are BP 92/58, PR 109 and temperature 38°. What should you do next?

a Further fluid challenge, arterial blood gas

b Put patient in head down tilt

c Catheterise

d All the above

With the information you have now gathered you try to contact your registrar and SHO. They are both in theatre, but say they will be done in an hour and a half. Two hours later the ward fast bleep you; when you arrive the patient is highly unresponsive, GCS 6/15. What airway adjunct would you use?

a Venturi mask 60%

b 15 L non-rebreathe bag and mask

c Laryngeal mask airway

d Guedel airway

As you are trying to bleep the SpR a nurse shouts for you to come over; the patient is now unresponsive and has arrested. You put out a crash call and start compressions. Once the gel pads are on the following rhythm is obtained:

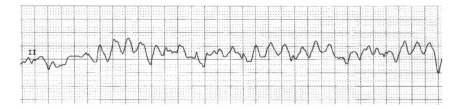

What is this rhythm?

a Ventricular tachycardia

b Atrial fibrillation

c Ventricular fibrillation

d Supraventricular tachycardia

What will be your next course of action?

a 150 J biphasic shock

b Adrenaline 1 mg IV

c Amiodarone 300 mg

d Continue chest compressions for a further 2 minutes

75 You are on call in the Emergency Department and you are referred a patient with a fractured neck of femur. On your initial assessment of the patient you note that he is drowsy and unresponsive to vocal commands. He is only making incomprehensible sounds. His temperature is 35.2°, respiratory rate is 34, pulse rate 140, BP 96/52 and oxygen saturations are 80% on room air. A quick inspection shows his airway to be clear. You note that he has orange discolouration of his right index and middle fingers.

What action would you take first to resuscitate this patient?

a   Oxygen 15 litres per minute, via non-rebreathe bag and mask

b   Oxygen at 28% via Venturi mask

c   1 litre of Hartmann's solution stat

d   Intubate and ventilate

After administering the above treatment, you take an arterial blood gas and it reveals a pH of 7.1, pCO_2 11.6 kPa, pO_2 17.2 kPa, HCO_3^- 33. What does this represent?

a   Metabolic acidosis

b   Respiratory acidosis

c   Respiratory alkalosis

d   Normal ABG

Which of the answers below is the most likely diagnosis?

a   Septic arthritis

b   Acute haemorrhage

c   Pulmonary oedema

d   Infective exacerbation of COPD

Answers

1 b, a, b, e

The principle differentials for this male child are acute appendicitis and mesenteric adenitis (inflammation of the mesenteric lymph nodes). It is, however, important to note that the two can coexist. If the patient was female then gynaecological causes should be sought, e.g. ectopic pregnancy, acute salpingitis, or ruptured ovarian cyst. Mesenteric adenitis is most frequently caused by viral pathogens, which would be indicated by a raised lymphocyte count, whereas a raised neutrophil count would suggest a bacterial origin. *Campylobacter*, *Salmonella*, and *Shigella* can all cause gastroenteritis that can mimic appendicitis, however vomiting usually precedes any colic.

The history of coryzal symptoms raises the question of mesenteric adenitis, and as such an ultrasound scan (USS) may be useful in identifying features such as enlarged lymph nodes or abnormal appendix. With the clinical suspicion being mesenteric adenitis, and imaging to support this, close monitoring would be acceptable (provided the patient is stable) before undertaking an operation.

2   a, c, b, c

From the history of ulcerative colitis with adenocarcinoma it is likely this lady has undergone a total proctocolectomy. This is supported by the stoma on the right hand side, which is likely to be an end ileostomy, especially as the primary procedure was an emergency.

The description given is that of subacute bowel obstruction and this is likely to be secondary to adhesions. The swelling upon raising the head may make you think that this could be strangulated however from the examination findings this is likely to be a large necked, easily reducible parastomal hernia containing small bowel.

The appropriate management of this patient would be to initiate intravenous fluids to replace lost volume and decompress the stomach with a nasogastric (NG) tube (drip and suck). If the patient does not settle, symptoms progress, distension worsens, or the observations change (e.g. pulse rate becomes greater than the systolic BP), then urgent operative intervention will be necessary.

3 a, c, e, c

This gentleman has two principle causes for his epigastric pain to narrow down the differential diagnosis; he is a publican and therefore could have a greater consumption of alcohol than most and he has recently increased his dose of voltarol (diclofenac) which is a non-steroidal anti-inflammatory drug (NSAID). He is also described as being overweight; his ECG shows non-specific changes in the inferior leads, so reference to previous ECGs, together with cardiac enzymes would be indicated to exclude myocardial infarction.

The history is more likely to be that of peptic ulcer disease secondary to NSAIDs. To prove the diagnosis and to rule out a malignancy an endoscopy would be appropriate. Aside from NSAIDs, *Helicobacter pylori*, a *Campylobacter*-like organism (hence CLO test), is a common cause of ulceration. This Gram –ve motile rod, has potent urease activity leading to the formation of ammonia and this neutralises the pH causing increased secretion of HCl. Many strains also produce cytokines that possess protease and phospholipase activity allowing them to attach to mucosal membranes. Treatment is with triple therapy, typically a proton pump inhibitor, i.e. lansoprazole, and two antibiotics: amoxicillin and clarithromycin.

4 b, b, e, a

The history contains the classic 4 F's:

- Fat
- Female
- Fertile
- Forty

A likely diagnosis is gallstone disease. This patient is currently stable, however if a stone was to pass into the common bile duct (CBD) causing subsequent bile outflow obstruction then there is a risk of gallstone pancreatitis or, if an infection develops, ascending cholangitis.

The most appropriate treatment would be a laparoscopic cholecystectomy. An on table cholangiogram would only be performed if there were suspicion of stones in the CBD, CBD stricture or damage to the CBD.

Gallstone ileus is when a stone ulcerates through the gall bladder wall into the duodenum and impacts on the narrowest part of the small bowel, i.e. the ileocaecal valve (ileus is actually a misnomer as it is a mechanical obstruction). A key feature is gas in the biliary tree, which can be seen on a plain abdominal film.

The prevalence of stones is approximately 75% mixed, 20% cholesterol, 5% bile pigment. Lecithin (a phospholipid) is a subliming agent. It is a relative decrease in this that can lead to the formation of gallstones. Calcium oxalate is the most common constituent of renal calculi.

5 b, e, a, b

Cellulitis and deep vein thrombosis are likely to be the top differentials; deep vein thrombosis is a little more likely as the patient has had major abdominal surgery with a likely period of immobility postoperatively. Before starting treatment it is important to take blood cultures and mark the outline of the erythematous area with indelible ink. As the suspicion of both has been raised, it is important to treat and ensure that doses are given in the A&E department. An urgent Doppler ultrasound should be arranged for that day and treatment adjusted accordingly.

Virchow's triad outlines the precipitating factors of intraluminal thrombus formation, these being stasis, hypercoagulability and endothelial damage. Virchow's node describes the supraclavicular lymph nodes, and when enlarged in gastric carcinoma is described as Troisier's sign. Option c) describes the 3 D's of pellagra, vitamin B3 deficiency. Option d) describes Meniere's disease. Option e) makes up the landmarks of the cystic artery as described by Calot.

6 b, b, e, a

This gentleman demonstrates the 6 P's of acute ischaemia:

- Pain
- Pallor
- Pulseless
- Perishingly cold
- Pareasthesia
- Paralysis

Ankle brachial pressure index (ABPI) should be recorded. This is done by using a Doppler probe and BP cuff to measure the systolic pressure at which the brachial and dorsalis pedis pulses become undetectable using the probe. The ratio between the two is then calculated by dividing the DP pulse pressure by the brachial pulse pressure. Ischaemia warranting urgent surgical intervention is said to be present if the ratio is less than 0.5.

With Buerger's test the feet reperfuse with a dusky crimson colour in contrast to a normally perfused foot, which has no colour change.

Given that this gentleman has critical leg ischaemia of recent onset, the most appropriate management would be an urgent embolectomy to restore blood supply to the ischaemic limb.

The patient gives a history of intermittent claudication and is therefore likely to be an arteriopath; this increases his risk for a myocardial infarction due to atherosclerosis and subsequent thrombus formation in the coronary arteries.

7   a, b, e, d

An aneurysm is an abnormal permanent dilatation of an artery. The most severe complication of an aortic aneurysm is rupture, which is around 5% per annum once the diameter is ≥ 6 cm. Operative mortality is 3–7% and so it is at 5.5 cm diameter that a decision to repair should be made, based on the patient's wishes, anatomical relations of the aneurysm and comorbidities.

Aneurysms of 4 cm in diameter should be monitored with ultrasound scans every 6/12. Plethysmography is a non-invasive method of measuring blood flow and is not used for the surveillance of abdominal aortic aneurysms (AAA). At the time of writing, a national screening programme for AAA using abdominal ultrasound scans in all men over the age of 65 years was under consideration by each of the four UK health departments.

Medial degenerative disease refers to breakdown of varying degrees of the tunica media of the artery in question; this leads to a decrease in the tensile strength of the arterial wall and therefore increases the risk of aneurysm. Aventitial inflammation and subsequent fibrosis is thought to weaken the vessel wall, again making an aneurysm more likely. A *Salmonella* bacteraemia can cause infection of an existing atherosclerotic plaque and weaken the artery from the luminal surface. Connective tissue disorders (e.g. Marfan's syndrome) result in a tunica media that has reduced tolerance to shear stresses caused by high pressure blood flow in the great vessels; these patients are therefore at increased aneurysm risk.

Endovascular aneurysm repair (EVAR) is becoming increasingly more common, with a prosthetic graft positioned at the site of the aneurysm by introducing it through the femoral artery.

8   a, e, c, a

Venous ulcers, which account for 90% of all ulcers, commonly occur around the malleoli. It is possible to differentiate venous disease from other causes of ulceration from the history and examination. Ischaemic/arterial ulceration will have the findings listed in B, with the limb being cool to touch and a low ABPI (ankle brachial pressure index). Neuropathic ulceration, commonly associated with diabetes, will lack sensation in the surrounding area. A malignant ulcer, particularly squamous carcinoma, may arise from a pre-existing chronic ulcer (Marjolin's ulcer), meaning surveillance is important. Ulcerated malignant melanoma is another cause of neoplastic ulcer. Systemic disease, e.g. ulcerative colitis, must also be thought of.

Venous ulcers have a ragged edge, an area of advancing epithelium that may appear as a blue rim. The ulceration is caused in this case by venous hypertension, likely due to incompetent deep veins. This generates high resting pressures and results in fluid transudation, oedema and poor skin nutrition.

The most appropriate treatment, as the history and examination findings indicate a non-infected venous ulcer, is compression bandaging after measurement of ABPI to ensure that there is no arterial insufficiency. Antibiotics are only considered if the ulcer is grossly infected with surrounding cellulitis.

Trendelenburg's test detects reflux from deep to superficial veins and can identify the site of the incompetent valves by placement of the tourniquet. Lachman's tests for anterior cruciate ligament injuries with the knee at 15–20° flexion.

9   c, a, a, a

The history indicates a probable head of pancreas carcinoma. The history and examination findings describe Courvoisier's law, which states 'if in the presence of jaundice the gallbladder is palpable then the jaundice is unlikely to be due to stone'.

Murphy's sign is guarding in the right upper quadrant (RUQ) upon deep inspiration. Rovsing's sign is when palpation of the left iliac fossa causes greater pain on the right. Trousseau's sign is thrombophlebitis migrans associated with pancreatic carcinoma. Homans' sign is positive if passive dorsiflexion of the foot elicits pain in the ipsilateral calf, a sign of deep vein thrombosis.

Ca 19-9 is a tumour marker grossly raised in pancreatic carcinoma. It can also be raised with other pathology but not to such a great extent, e.g. colorectal carcinoma, gastric carcinoma and hepatoma. Ca 125 is specific for ovarian carcinoma, Ca 15-3 is raised in breast cancer, AFP (α-fetoprotein) is raised in the presence of hepatocellular carcinoma or teratoma, and CEA (carcinoembryonic antigen) is used to monitor recurrence of colorectal carcinoma postoperatively.

Adenocarcinoma is the most common pancreatic cancer. Gastrinoma and insulinoma can occur but have a different symptom set. Gastrinoma (Zollinger-Ellison syndrome) typically presents with upper gastrointestinal bleeding or perforation and multiple duodenal ulcers due to the secretion of gastrin-like substance and subsequent high levels of HCl. Insulinoma patients present with Whipple's triad of:

- Attacks of fainting or muscle weakness induced by exercise or starvation.
- Hypoglycaemia.
- Symptoms relieved by dextrose given orally or intravenously.

A curative procedure is only possible if the cancer is confined to the peri-ampullary region. A Whipple's procedure, pancreaticoduodenectomy, removes part of the duodenum, the pancreatic head, common bile duct, followed by formation of a gastroenterostomy and biliary drainage using a Roux loop of jejunum to restore continuity.

10 a, c, b, a

From the history this patient would have undergone coronary artery bypass grafting (CABG). The scar described is a midline sternotomy. A thoracotomy scar runs obliquely around the patient's chest wall, crossing the mid-axilliary line and extending posteriorly. A Lanz incision is used for a muscle dividing appendectomy; laparotomy is a midline longitudinal incision that gives good access to the abdominal cavity and is used for many operations, and a Kocher incision is for open cholecystectomy.

The vein that runs on the medial aspect of the leg is the long saphenous vein, which originates from where the dorsal vein of the first digit (the large toe) merges with the dorsal venous arch of the foot, passing anterior to the medial malleolus and draining into the femoral vein at the saphenofemoral junction. This is a common vein used for CABG; other vessels include the internal mammary artery or the radial artery. Primary and rescue percutaneous intervention (PCI) has largely replaced the need for CABG; however for total occlusion, severe left main stem disease, or extensive multivessel disease not amenable to PCI, CABG is still indicated.

Medical therapy has come a long way over recent years, though remains less successful than both PCI and CABG in the management of myocardial infarction. Clopidogrel is an ADP (adenosine diphosphate) inhibitor. This then prevents the binding of ADP to its receptor and subsequent activation of the glycoprotein GPIIb/IIIa complex. Anti Xa is the site of the low molecular weight heparins (LMWH), e.g. enoxaparin. GPIIb/IIIa inhibitors prevent the final common pathway of platelet aggregation, e.g. abciximab, tirofiban. These mediators are useful to be considered in patients who are diagnosed early and if PCI is to be undertaken. GTN should be given to all patients suffering from stable angina or acute coronary syndrome (ACS).

11 b, d, c, c

Clean operations are those elective cases in which the gastrointestinal (GI) tract or respiratory tract is not entered; clean contaminated are elective cases in which the GI tract or respiratory tract is entered but there is no gross spillage of contents; contaminated are those in which a fresh traumatic wound is present or gross spillage of GI contents occurs; dirty operations include those in which bacterial inflammation or pus is present.

A useful system is to divide operative complications into immediate, early, late, local and systemic. The likely source of this patient's swinging pyrexia, with tender abdomen, is a collection.

A quick mnemonic for postoperative pyrexia is the 7 C's:

- Cut (wound)
- Collection
- Chest (atelectasis/pneumonia)
- Catheter (UTI)
- Cannula (superficial thrombophlebitis)
- Central line
- Calf (deep vein thrombosis)

Patients are susceptible to infection while in hospital for a number of reasons, some of the most concerning and certainly most publicised infections are the antibiotic resistant strains, i.e. methicillin-resistant *Staph. aureas* (MRSA) and extended spectrum β-lactamase (ESBL*)*. *Clostridium difficile*, a toxin producing Gram +ve anaerobic spore forming bacteria, usually occurs in patients who have received broad-spectrum antibiotics, in this case cefuroxime. The 027 strain is particularly troublesome as it produces more toxins and is associated with increased mortality and more relapses. If the patient is suspected to have *C. diff.* then they must be isolated and stool samples sent for *C. diff.* toxin and usual microscopy culture and sensitivity. First line treatment after adequate fluid and electrolyte replacement is oral metronidazole then oral vancomycin. In particularly resistant cases, where the patient is unlikely to contract TB, rifampicin may also be used in concert with local microbiology advice.

12 d, a, e, c

Hidradenitis suppurativa is due to the infection of apocrine sweat glands, particularly of the axillae and groin. They do not respond to antimicrobial therapy and can only really be treated effectively by excision of the affected skin. Conservative measures will include improving personal hygiene and hexachlorophene baths.

A furuncle is an abscess with a single drainage point, which involves a follicle and its associated glands, whereas a carbuncle has multiple drainage points. Both are staphylococcal in origin.

A pilonidal abscess occurs in the natal cleft. The main theory on the mechanism of formation is that a hair works its way into a follicle due to its tapered end. This then causes a foreign body reaction and produces a chronic infected sinus. Treatment is to excise the sinus after exploration, or lay it open and allow to heal by granulation tissue. Removing of hair locally postoperatively may reduce recurrence.

A sebaceous cyst most commonly presents around the scalp, ears, back, face and upper arm, though may occur anywhere. It is characterised by a central punctum. Its origin is a sebaceous gland in the epidermis and is caused by blocked sebaceous glands and a high testosterone level. It contains sebum, produced by the gland. These cysts do not usually require surgical intervention unless they become infected or painful, or there are cosmetic reasons.

All these forms of local skin excision are prone to scarring and recurrence postoperatively and patients must be made aware of this at the time of consent.

13 b, a, a, a

This is the classic history of an extradural haematoma with temporary concussion followed by initial recovery (the lucid interval). There then follows a deterioration in consciousness level over a period of several hours due to cerebral compression by the growing extradural clot. Alternatively the patient can become progressively worse with no lucid interval.

On examination there maybe localising signs such as pupil dilatation, indicating the side of the haematoma, however 10% will have false localising signs and a degree of high vigilance is needed. The patient should, once stable, proceed to urgent CT scanning. An extradural haematoma generally causes a convex (and subdural a concave/crescent) shaped opacity on the CT scan. Acute subdural haematoma usually results from a severe head injury and the patient deteriorates from the moment of trauma. CT is the most useful investigation. Subgaleal haematoma is formed under the subaponeurotic layer of the scalp.

A subarachnoid haemorrhage is bleeding in the subarachnoid space (between the arachnoid membrane and the pia mater). It has a classic presentation of 'thunderclap headache' – this is described as a sudden-onset very severe headache, as if being struck on the top of the head. It is often caused by an intracranial vessel rupture, for example from a Berry aneurysm. It carries a poor prognosis; the mortality on the initial hospital admission alone is around 50%.

The Glasgow Coma Score is calculated as follows:

TABLE 1: Glasgow Coma Score

Eye opening (E)	Verbal response (V)	Motor response (M)
4 = Spontaneous	5 = Normal conversation	6 = Normal
3 = To voice	4 = Disoriented conversation	5 = Localises to pain
2 = To pain		4 = Withdraws to pain
1 = None	3 = Words, but not coherent	3 = Decorticate posture
	2 = Incomprehensible sounds	2 = Decerebrate
		1 = None
	1 = None	

If the patient is intubated then the score is out of 10.

14 a, a, b, b

This describes amaurosis fugax, a transient monocular visual loss. A cerebrovascular infarct or haemorrhage (stroke) is likely to result in weakness of the contralateral side to which the event occurred. If the dominant hemisphere is involved speech may be affected. A transient ischaemic attack is similar in signs and symptoms, however the symptoms fully resolve within 24 hours.

Duplex ultrasound is a useful non-invasive first line investigation if stenosis is seen; this can be further characterised by magnetic resonance angiography (MRA) or normal angiography. Angiography is not without risk and a thrombus can be dislodged precipitating an embolic stroke.

Carotid endarterectomy of asymptomatic stenosis may be undertaken provided the risk benefit ratio is acceptable. Patients who are symptomatic and with > 70% stenosis will require endarterectomy in which the diseased intima is removed while a preoperative shunt is used to maintain blood flow.

The complications to this surgery are serious, with up to 5% of patients suffering a stroke. This patient is exhibiting hypoglossal neuropraxia, due to the hypoglossal nerve crossing the upper part of the incision, and so has been damaged during the surgery. Reperfusion syndrome can also occur due to the sudden increase in blood flow resulting in oedema and fitting. This is prevented by good postoperative BP control.

15 a, c, c, e

Basal skull fractures are relatively rare isolated findings, with just 4% as an isolated fracture in severe head injury. The presence of CSF is pathognomonic of this fracture. Raccoon or panda eyes are bilateral haemorrhages into the soft tissue around the eyes. Bruising over the suboccipital region or mastoid process is known as Battle's sign. Grey-Turner's and Cullen's signs are seen as a result of severe pancreatitis.

A nasopharyngeal (NP) airway should be avoided due to the potential risk of inserting it through the fracture and into the cranial vault. In this case an oral airway is preferred. NP airways are made of soft malleable plastic, bevelled at one end with a flange at the other. It is better tolerated than oropharyngeal airways in those patients that are not deeply unconscious.

The symptoms described form part of Beck's triad of cardiac tamponade:

- Hypotension due to decreased stroke volume.

- Jugular venous distension due to impaired venous return to the heart.

- Muffled heart sounds due to fluid inside the pericardium.

Tamponade occurs when there is rapid filling of the pericardial sac, i.e. due to trauma. This compresses the heart and can lead to obstructive cardiogenic shock. Treatment involves draining the effusion (pericardiocentesis) while the patient is connected to a cardiac monitor to check for electrical disturbance, which may typically occur if the needle is inserted too far and touches the myocardium.

16 b, b, d, a

Carpal tunnel syndrome (CTS) is a compressive neuropathy of the median nerve at the wrist. Carpal tunnel syndrome may be caused by repetitive manual work (though this is controversial), pregnancy, hypothyroidism, acromegaly, local trauma and neoplasia. The carpal tunnel is formed by the flexor retinaculum stretching from the hook of the hamate and pisiform medially to the trapezium and scaphoid laterally. This leads to wasting of the thenar eminence, diminished sensation and pain.

Two clinical tests used to examine the patient with suspected CTS are Tinel's, in which tapping the volar wrist over the median nerve may produce paraesthesia in the median distribution of the hand, and Phalen's test, as described in the question. Chvostek's sign is positive if tapping over the facial nerve, about 2 cm anterior to the tragus of the ear, causes twitching of the facial muscles. Trousseau's sign is positive if inflation of a BP cuff above the systolic causes local ulnar and median nerve ischaemia resulting in carpal spasm. Both are clinical signs of hypocalcaemia. Uhthoff's phenomenon is described in patients with demyelinating disease such as multiple sclerosis; an increase in detected temperature, either on exercise or caused by an external heat source, causes a temporary worsening of neurological symptoms, typically worsening of vision.

Diagnosis is confirmed by nerve conduction studies. The concern with CTS is that the nerve may become permanently damaged. This case is not severe and there is a potential for reversal of symptoms after delivery; reassurance and review are all that is needed. Further treatment may be indicated if symptoms persist or worsen after delivery; an elective decompression might then be appropriate treatment.

17 e, a, b, d

Rupture at oesophagealogastroduodenoscopy (OGD) is usually at the level of the cricopharyngeus or above a stricture. Spontaneous rupture of the oesophagus occurs rarely and is associated with vomiting (Boerhaave's syndrome). A Mallory-Weiss tear is associated with upper gastrointestinal bleed as a result of repetitive vomiting causing a longitudinal mucosal laceration without perforation. Plummer-Vinson syndrome is dysphasia, caused by an oesophageal web and iron deficiency anaemia. The condition is premalignant and is associated with the development of a carcinoma in cricopharyngeal region.

A gastrograffin (water-soluble contrast) swallow will confirm a perforation and define its position. A plain chest radiograph (not offered in the question) may show gas in the neck and mediastinum. The treatment option for cervical perforation is with parenteral antibiotics, patient nil by mouth and adequate fluid resuscitation. If the thoracic oesophagus had been ruptured then surgery would be needed. Abscess formation in the superior mediastinum requires drainage via a supraclavicular incision.

18 d, a, a, a

Acute gastric erosions secondary to non-steroidal use are common – in this case diclofenac. While oesophageal varices will be in the differential diagnosis, his observations are stable. First the patient must be resuscitated; after ensuring that the patient's airway is secure and that there is no compromise of breathing or lung function, two large bore cannulae are inserted in each antecubital fossa, with blood taken for group and save, haemoglobin and clotting studies. IV fluids should be commenced. Once the patient has been adequately resuscitated and is stable, OGD should be considered to either confirm the diagnosis, rule out *Campylobacter* infection or malignancy.

TABLE 2: Rockall Scoring System

Variable	Risk score			
	0	1	2	3
Age (years)	< 60	60–79	> 79	–
Shock	BP > 100 mm, Hg pulse < 100 bpm	BP > 100 mm, Hg pulse > 100 bpm	BP < 100 mm, Hg pulse > 100 bpm	–
Comorbidity	None	–	Cardiac disease, any other major comorbidity	Renal failure, liver failure, disseminated malignancy
Endoscopic diagnosis	Mallory-Weiss tear, no lesion	All other diagnoses	Malignancy of the upper GI tract	–
Major SRH	None, or dark spots	–	Blood in the upper GI tract, adherent clot or spurting vessel	–

Key:
BP = blood pressure; GI = gastrointestinal; SRH = stigmata of recent haemorrhage.

TABLE 3: Rebleed and mortality risk according to Rockall score

Risk score	Predicted rebleed (%)	Predicted mortality (%)
0	5	0
1	3	0
2	5	0
3	11	3
4	14	5
5	24	11
6	33	17
7	44	27
8+	42	41

Aside form the CLO test, *H. pylori* can be diagnosed using carbon 13 urea breath test. The patient is asked to drink a liquid containing urea that is labelled with carbon 13. Then the labelled carbon is measured on the patient's breath; this is only high when urease (as produced by *H. pylori*) is present in the stomach. Other tests include faecal antigen test that is used to detect eradication after treatment or serological testing based on the measurement of immunoglobulin to antibodies against *H. pylori*.

19 b, a, a, b

With a patient who is obstructed, the concern is that they either have or will have perforated their bowel releasing faecal material into the peritoneal cavity, thus causing generalised peritonitis. This is associated with considerable mortality. An erect chest radiograph (CXR) can be used to see if free air is present under the diaphragm. Complete constipation (obstipation) is the absence of passage of either flatus or faecal material.

A volvulus is the twisting of a loop of bowel around its mesenteric axis. A volvulus can also occur at the small intestine and rarely the stomach. It is relatively rare, accounting for 2% of intestinal obstruction and usually occurs in elderly constipated patients. If the patient is stable, a long rectal flatus tube is passed to the sigmoid colon; this often untwists early volvulus. If, however, this fails then laparotomy must be performed with the procedure dictated by the findings. In this case, where there is distended caecum with associated serosal tears, then the colon must be removed leaving the rectum intact and a stoma formed with a possibility for reversal at a later date. The fact that the small bowel is not dilated indicates that the ilio-caecal valve is intact.

20 a, a, c, a

Claudication of the cauda equina may arise as a result of lumbar canal stenosis. Symptoms are similar to those resulting from peripheral vascular disease with cramp-like leg pains, often associated with paraesthesia. Neurological claudication however worsens on standing, is relieved by sitting and the pulses are intact, whereas vascular claudication is usually unilateral, relieved on standing and peripheral pulses are diminished or absent.

The diagnosis is best made using MRI. While CT and plain lumbar radiographs are useful, MRI is the investigation of choice. Degenerative disc disease is a common cause of this claudication and osteophytes are described in the history, which would fit with the knowledge that he has osteoarthritis. The treatment can involve trial of conservative measures such as lumbar flexion exercises before surgical intervention is required.

Claudication is different to cauda equina syndrome, which is a neurosurgical emergency often warranting urgent surgical decompression. The red flags for this are saddle anaesthesia (over the buttocks, anus and perineum), weakness of the lower leg muscles, rapidly worsening neurological symptoms, absent ankle reflexes and urinary retention.

21 a, c, d, d

There are three main types of nerve injury:

1   Neuropraxia – damage to the nerve fibres, in which there is no disruption of the nerve or its sheath. The conduction is interrupted for only a short period of time, with recovery commencing soon after the injury and is complete in 6–8 weeks.

2   Axonotmesis – this is injury to the axon and myelin sheath without disruption of the continuity of its perineural sheath. The axon distal to the lesion degenerates, termed Wallerian degeneration, and this usually begins 24 hours after injury. The axonal skeleton disintegrates and the axonal membrane breaks apart; this is followed by degradation of the myelin sheath and macrophage infiltration. Regrowth in the axon occurs from the node of Ranvier proximal to the injury. The rate of regeneration is approximately 1 mm day^{-1}.

3   Neurotmesis – complete disruption of the nerve and nerve sheath. If the two ends are not too far displaced then regeneration may take place, however functional recovery will be incomplete.

EMG (electromyography) can be used in the assessment of nerve injury and in this case, where litigation may be an issue, it will be important to document EMG findings. The treatment of this patient will be to splint in the position of function and encourage regular passive movements, with physiotherapy input, to prevent immobility after the nerve has recovered.

22 b, b, c, a

Postgastrectomy syndromes include bilious vomiting, dumping syndrome, (which comprises of fainting and vertigo due to the high osmolarity of the gastric contents entering the jejunum absorbing fluid into the gut lumen and producing temporary reduction of circulating blood volume), steatorrhea, stomal ulceration and anaemia.

Removal of parietal cells will not only decrease acid secretion but also production of intrinsic factor. This is a glycoprotein that is necessary for B12 absorption through an ileal mucosa receptor specific for the B12-intrinsic factor complex that then enters the portal circulation.

I cells, which are located in the duodenum, produce cholecystokinin (CCK), which is responsible for stimulating the pancreas to secrete digestive enzymes. β-cells and δ-cells are pancreatic cells responsible for the production and secretion of insulin and glucagons respectively.

Pernicious anaemia is a form of megaloblastic anaemia in which auto-antibodies are directed against parietal cells and intrinsic factor. This can be diagnosed using Schilling's test. A drink containing radiolabelled B12 and an intramuscular injection of unlabelled B12 is given. The injection saturates stores therefore preventing the radiolabelled B12 being taken into tissue – it is instead excreted in the urine. The urine is then measured over the first 24 hours. A normal test shows at least 10% present in the urine; an abnormal test is less than 5%. If the test is abnormal it is repeated with oral intrinsic factor, if the B12 is then greater than 10% in the urine the diagnosis of pernicious anaemia can be made.

23 c, a, a, b

While iron tablets ($FeSO_4$) are a cause for black stools, there is nothing in the history to suggest this and a gastrointestinal bleed is likely. The patient should be resuscitated as necessary and a cause determined. A technetium-99 scan is the investigation of choice as it is taken up by gastric mucosa.

Meckel's diverticulum is the remnant of the vitello-intestinal duct, which usually undergoes complete obliteration during the seventh week of gestation. It typically lies on the antimesenteric border of the ileum and is said to:

- occur in 2% of the population
- be 2 feet (60 cm) from the ileocaecal valve
- average 2 inches (5 cm) in length
- be symptomatic in 2% of cases
- consist of two types of common ectopic tissue (gastric and pancreatic).

Treatment is surgical resection of the diverticulum.

24 c, c, e, c

Crohn's disease is a chronic transmural inflammatory process of the bowel that often leads to fibrosis and obstructive symptoms from the mouth to the anus. It is seen more frequently in smokers, in contrast to ulcerative colitis in which smoking appears to be protective. Patients with Crohn's disease most commonly present with symptoms related to chronic inflammatory process, such as low-grade fever, prolonged diarrhoea with abdominal pain and weight loss. The diarrhoea is usually non-bloody, with mucus and often intermittent. Patients may present with complaints suggestive of intestinal obstruction or extensive fistulating disease.

Barium studies can demonstrate cobble stoning as a result of tracking of deep ulceration both transversely and longitudinally, and small bowel strictures. CT can demonstrate mesenteric fat stranding caused by inflammation and MRI is useful at demonstrating complicated perianal fistula tracts.

Rigler's sign, positive when free air is present in the peritoneum, appears as air outlining the serosa of the bowel.

Conservative treatment for Crohn's is the cessation of smoking. Medical management remains the most effective treatment, however if this fails and uncontrolled disease occurs resulting in obstruction, then surgical treatment, i.e. resection is needed. Unlike ulcerative colitis, where a panproctocolectomy is curative, there is no cure.

25 a, d, b, b

Ovarian cancer typically causes minimal, non-specific or no symptoms in the early stages. Women present with vague abdominal/pelvic pain, bloating, distension and possible vaginal bleeding.

On examination the patient may have a palpable mass, ascites (as in this case) or a pleural effusion. The triad of ascites, pleural effusion (usually on the right side) and a benign ovarian tumour is known as Meigs' syndrome. If an ovarian cancer is suspected a Ca 125 should be requested. Imaging should be arranged, ideally CT staging involving the chest, abdomen and pelvis.

Ascites can be demonstrated clinically by shifting dullness or fluid thrill. This patient's ascites is the result of malignant exudates. The best way to discriminate between transudate and exudates is to use the serum ascites albumin gradient (SAAG) score. This is serum albumin concentration – ascitic albumin concentration. If > 1.1 g/dl the fluid is transudate, and if < 1.1 g/dl then an exudate. Transudates are a result of increased portal vein pressure, or lack of oncotic pressure, while exudates are actively secreted fluids, and are therefore high in protein. Exudates typically have a high LDH, a low pH and a low glucose.

26 c, b, d, a

Third spacing is non-recoverable fluid losses, e.g. the bowel lumen or peritoneum. This amount can be considerable in patients who are obstructed and accurate fluid balance and replacement is vital. Monitoring the central venous pressure is often very useful for monitoring the fluid status of a patient.

The mechanism of bowel perforation from obstruction is due to the local pressure of the obstructed faecal material on the bowel mucosa. This subsequently causes local ischaemia and local inflammation causing necrosis and perforation.

Adhesions from prior surgery account for 75% of all cases of small bowel obstruction. The period to obstruction can occur at any time from immediately postoperatively to many years later. It is important to note that large bowel obstruction is rarely due to adhesions.

The management of adhesions is initially conservative provided the patient is stable and not showing signs of perforation. A drip and suck regime is used; this involves insertion of a nasogastric tube for decompression and intravenous fluid for replacement. However, if the patient deteriorates or does not settle, then laparotomy with adhesiolysis or resection is warranted.

27 c, d, a, a

Carcinoid tumours are rare neuroendocrine lesions that arise from amine precursor uptake and decarboxylation cells (APUD cells). Common sites for primary tumours are appendix (30%) and small bowel (20%), however they may be found anywhere in the alimentary canal and also the lung.

They commonly secrete 5-hydroxytryptamine (5-HT, serotonin) but are rarely symptomatic until they have metastasised to the liver. In 10% of cases there is an association with multiple endocrine neoplasia type 1. Prior to metastasising, carcinoid tumours usually produce vague right sided abdominal discomfort, present for a number of years, and can result in bowel obstruction.

Once the tumour has metastasised (approx. 4%), patients may develop carcinoid syndrome. This comprises of flushing typically precipitated by stress or ingestion of food or alcohol. Other symptoms include diarrhoea, often profuse and tricuspid stenosis, although this is a late manifestation.

The diagnosis may be confirmed by increased 24-hour urinary 5-hydroxindole acetic acid. CT or USS may demonstrate an abdominal mass or live secondaries and radiolabelled octreotide scintography is useful to identify primary or secondary tumours. Treatment is by resection if caught early enough, both of primary disease and liver secondaries. Medical therapy can include somatostatin analogue that inhibits 5-HT release.

28 e, b, a

Diverticula are out-pouchings of the mucosal membrane through the muscle wall where the vasa recta penetrate the bowel, providing a mechanically weak point. They are lined solely by mucosa and are therefore defined as false diverticular due to the lack of normal muscle layer, unlike a Meckel's diverticulum, which is a true diverticulum. The pathogenesis that has been proposed is due to the low residue diet in the West; high intraluminal pressures are needed to propel the stool and this in turn causes herniation of the mucosa at the sites of potential weakness in the bowel wall.

Diverticuli can occur anywhere in the gastrointestinal tract, but are usually seen in the colon, particularly sigmoid and descending colon. These diverticuli can become infected – diverticulitis can lead to complications. They may perforate, causing abscess formation, fistula formation (as with this patient) or frank peritonitis, a life threatening condition. They can produce chronic infection and inflammation leading to stricture formation and obstruction. Vessel erosion can occur, causing haemorrhage to varying degrees.

Colovesical fistula is often given away in the history by passage of gas bubbles (pneumaturia) and faecal debris in the urine. There may also be a history of recurrent urinary tract infections. On CT scan gas can be seen in the bladder; the fistula may be better demonstrated on a water-soluble contrast enema. Treatment is by resection of the affected segment of colon and bladder, with a covering loop ileostomy to protect the anastomosis, which can later be reversed.

29 a, a, c, a

Femoral hernias are more common in females, however inguinal hernias are still more frequent than femoral. The boundaries of the femoral canal are:

- anteriorly: the inguinal ligament
- medially: the sharp edge of the lacunar part of the inguinal ligament
- laterally: the femoral vein
- posteriorly: the pectineal ligament.

The neck of the femoral hernia lies below and lateral to the pubic tubercle, unlike an indirect inguinal hernia which extends above and medial to this landmark. The neck of the femoral canal is narrow; this can make irreducibility and strangulation common.

Richter's hernia is particularly common in the femoral sac, and is where only part of the wall rather than the whole bowel herniates through the defect. Due to the bowel lumen not being disrupted, obstructive symptoms do not occur. The risk of strangulation and therefore compromise of the vascular supply causing necrosis and perforation is high and the hernia will need repair.

Spigelian hernias pass through the arcuate line lateral to the rectus abdominis. They present as a tender mass to one side of the lower abdominal wall.

30 b, e, c, d

Hiatal hernias are of two common types: sliding (90%) and rolling (10%). Sliding is when the stomach 'slides' through the diaphragmatic hiatus, causing disturbance of the cardioesophageal sphincter. Rolling hernias have a portion of the stomach that 'rolls' up anteriorly to the oesophagus, but due to the cardioesophageal sphincter remaining intact these patients do not have reflux symptoms. The clinical features are predominantly reflux related with epigastric discomfort being common, particularly after lying down. This can lead to oesophageal stricture formation and bleeding in severe cases.

Divarification of the rectus abdominis muscles presents as the presence of a midline abdominal mass on raising the intra-abdominal pressure, e.g. on sitting up from a supine position. The condition is painless and there is little risk of bowel obstruction. The condition often presents in patients who are unfit and overweight. Conservative management is indicated for this.

The patients tend to be obese and so treatment should be aimed at lifestyle changes and antacids, proton pump inhibitors can be used for symptom relief. Rolling hernias do have the potential for complete volvulus and may require urgent surgical repair.

The vena cava passes through the diaphragm at T8 (vena cava has 8 letters), the aorta at T12, and the oesophagus at T10. The umbilicus is L4-L5 with the aorta bifurcating at L4 and the inferior vena cava at L5.

31 a, b, d

Rectal bleeding should always raise suspicion. This is a young patient with no 'red flags'; the main differentials are those listed in the question. Fissure-in-ano is a tear at the anal margin and usually the patient will report straining at defecation. The bleeding is local, bright red in nature and not mixed with the stool. Pain is stinging in nature and lasts for a while after the passage of stool. This pain worsens the constipation as the patient avoids going to the toilet in an effort to prevent the pain. On examination it may be possible to see the fissure, proctoscopy and rigid sigmoidoscopy may not be tolerated without anaesthetic. Chronic fissures can be seen with a sentinel pile and hypertrophic anal papillae.

Treatment will initially involve, alongside stool softeners and dietary advice, an ointment that relaxes the anal internal sphincter (under involuntary control), allowing the epithelium to heal. As this patient suffers from migraines the sensible option is to use 2% diltiazem cream BD topically. If this fails then the next step is to use botulinum toxin injection into the internal sphincter, the theory being this gives a more sustained effect than topical ointments. If this fails then an anal advancement flap to cover a freshened fissure would be considered. In some centres, injection of a fibrin/collagen matrix into the fissure may also be considered.

32 a, d, e, c

A fistula is an abnormal communication between two epithelial surfaces. Fistula-in-ano can occur as a consequence of an infection in the anal glands, the resulting pus formed then tracts through the soft tissue to form a fistula tract. Other causes must be excluded: Crohn's disease (particularly in this case), ulcerative colitis and rectal cancer. Fistulae can be classified by their relationship to the anatomy: suprasphincteric, transphincteric, intersphincteric and superficial. The course of the tract is variable. If the patient is in the lithotomy position (supine with legs up) a horizontal line can be imagined running at the level of the anus; if the external opening is posterior to the line then the internal opening is in the midline; if the external opening is anterior to this line then the internal opening is usually in line. This is Goodsall's rule, though it is not predictive 100% of the time.

Patients with perianal haematoma typically present to A&E with severe pain after straining. The pea sized exquisitely tender mass is usually just at the anal margin but with no mucosa, as it is covered with squamous epithelium supplied by somatic nerves explaining the pain. Great relief is achieved after an injection of local anaesthetic and the haematoma evacuated.

33 c, a, d, e

Patients with a history of rectal bleeding should be asked about the red flags that would indicate a possible malignancy:

- age
- dark/altered blood
- blood mixed in the stools
- incomplete emptying of the bowels (tenesmus)
- weight loss
- change in bowel habit
- loss of appetite
- lethargy
- significant family history
- palpable abdominal mass
- palpable rectal mass.

Haemorrhoids are congested vascular cushions, which under normal circumstances are involved in the continence mechanism. They usually occur following straining when passing stool and are traumatised by the passage of hard stool.

Their location is described when the patient is in lithotomy position and is usually at 3, 7 and 11 o'clock. They are graded on their appearance and degree of prolapse:

- 1st degree: confined to the anal canal
- 2nd degree: prolapse on defecation then spontaneously reduce
- 3rd degree: remain prolapsed and may require digital replacement.

34 b, b, a, d

This patient has painless jaundice. Courvoisier's law states 'if in the presence of jaundice the gall bladder is palpable, then the jaundice is unlikely to be due to a stone'. It is therefore likely that this patient has head of pancreas carcinoma, which accounts for 60% of pancreatic tumours.

This patient is jaundiced due to posthepatic obstruction. This means that while the bilirubin is conjugated by the liver, it cannot be excreted. Without the pigment from the bilirubin stools appear pale with conjugated bilirubin accumulating in the blood. This is renally excreted turning the urine dark brown. Other posthepatic causes must ruled out. The common bile duct is essentially a tube and the ways in which it can be blocked can be thought of as:

- inside the lumen: gallstones
- within the tube wall: stricture
                          sclerosing cholangitis
                          cholangiocarcinoma
- external compression: head of pancreas tumour
                          ampulla of Vater tumour.

35 c, b, d, a

The history implies alcohol misuse. If this is severe, liver cirrhosis may result, which can cause portal hypertension, hepatocellular failure and possible malignant change. The worsening abdominal distension this patient is experiencing is likely to be the accumulation of ascitic fluid, which is a combination of hypoalbuminaemia and portal hypertension. This occurs due to hepatocellular damage and thus a reduction in hepatic synthetic function (e.g. albumin and clotting factors) and an increased vascular resistance to blood flow from the portal venous system.

Portal hypertension (> 15 cm H_2O) can cause collateral formation, importantly left gastric vein to oesophageal vein, forming varices and to a lesser extent the other collaterals listed in the question stem. Splenomegaly occurs due to portal congestion and can be associated with leucopaenia and thrombocytopaenia as a result of hypersplenism.

A large volume of ascites or any large mass within the abdominal cavity can splint the diaphragm and cause difficulty in breathing. The most effective initial treatment is to remove the ascites by paracentesis followed by the use of diuretics, first line being spironolactone.

Pickwickian syndrome is hypoxia and hypercapnia as a result of severe obesity causing difficulty in respiration leading to daytime somnolence (type II respiratory failure).

36 e, d, b, c

This patient is suffering from severe pancreatitis and is already on ITU for close monitoring and system support. The causes of pancreatitis and the first two of the mnemonic GET SMASHED are the most common, i.e. gallstones and ethanol.

After such an insult on the pancreas, an inflammatory process results and causes proenzymes that normally do not damage the pancreatic tissue to leak out and become activated. This leads to widespread autodigestion not only confined to the pancreas. If this continues then liquefying necrotic material and inflammatory exudates collect in the lesser sac, a pseudocyst because of the absence of an epithelial layer.

Grey-Turner's sign develops from extravasation of blood-stained pancreatic juice into retroperitoneal fluid. Amylase, while significantly raised in the acute phase and useful to aid diagnosis, is not part of the Glasgow or Ranson criteria. The mnemonic PANCREAS is useful to remember these key scoring points for the Glasgow score.

- $PaO_2 < 8\,kPa$
- Age > 55 years
- N (neutrophils) white cell count > 15
- Calcium < 2.0
- Renal urea > 16
- Enzymes: AST > 200, LDH > 600
- Albumin < 32
- Sugar glucose > 10

A gastrinoma is a tumour that secretes gastrin, a hormone that is normally produced by G cells in the stomach and duodenum. Gastrin stimulates the secretion of gastric acid by the parietal cells in the stomach. An excess of gastrin (Zollinger-Ellison syndrome) leads to peptic ulcers in approximately 95% of patients with the syndrome. A gastrinoma is most commonly located in the duodenum or the pancreas.

37 e, b, c, a

Sickle cell anaemia is an autosomal recessive disease that results from the substitution of valine for glutamic acid, leaving a defective form of haemoglobin (HbS). It is deoxygenation of these that causes the classic sickle shape. The life span of a sickle cell is 10–20 days compared to the normal 120 days and can result in a prehepatic jaundice due to the release of unconjugated bilirubin in cell breakdown.

Acute splenic sequestration in which sickled cells block splenic out-flow leads to the pooling of peripheral blood in the engorged spleen causing splenomegaly. Splenectomy may be advocated in older children who have experienced splenic sequestration.

Postoperatively the platelet count rises but will subsequently settle; during this time there is a greater risk of developing a deep vein thrombosis and pulmonary embolus, so appropriate prophylaxis must be given. Due to the role of the spleen in removing capsulated micro-organisms, e.g. *Strep. pneumonia, Haemophilus influenzae* and *Neisseria meningitides*. Pneumovax and meningococcal vaccines are given along with prophylactic daily dose antibiotics typically for 2 years in adults.

38 a, b, a, a

Typically 20% of gallstones are cholesterol, 5% are bile pigment and 73% mixed. Only 10% of gallstones are visible on plain radiograph, while 90% of ureteric stones are radio opaque.

Fat soluble vitamins are A, D, E and K.

In the bowel lumen, bilirubin is reduced to urobilinogen by bacteria. Most of this is re-excreted as urobilirubin; a small amount of urobilinogen is reabsorbed from the terminal ileum into the portal venous system and returns to the liver. Here it is either excreted again back into the gut or a small amount reaches systemic circulation and is renally excreted.

39 c, b, c, e

Testicular tumours are the commonest solid malignancy in young adult men. Undescended and ectopic testis is associated with a 7× risk of developing a testicular tumour. The two main types are seminoma and non-seminomatous germ cell tumours. Lymphatic spread is to the para-aortic node due to the lymphatic vessels accompanying the testicular vein. In advanced cases the supraclavicular nodes may be involved.

The second case describes testicular torsion, a urological emergency and must be differentiated from other complaints of testicular pain because a delay can lead to loss of the testicle. After a 24-hour period of torsion there is little chance of salvaging the testicle. The testicle is covered by the tunica vaginalis; this attaches to the postero-lateral surface of the testicle and allows little mobility. In patients who have inappropriately high attachment the testicle can rotate freely which can cause compromise of the testicular artery.

Testicular torsion is a clinical diagnosis and imaging studies usually are not indicated as they simply delay definitive treatment. Initial management should be to try and attempt manual detorsion, achieved by untwisting the testicle from the midline out. The patient will still need urgent scrotal exploration.

40 b, a, a, a

Mastalgia can be divided into cyclical and non-cyclical. Non-cyclical breast pain can include: carcinoma of the breast, although this is an uncommon presenting symptom; an abscess; a chest wall lesion; Tietze's syndrome. Tietze's syndrome, a diagnosis of exclusion, is chostochondritis of unknown cause and usually resolves over a number of months.

Traumatic fat necrosis is typically associated with seat belt injury or trauma. It can be difficult to differentiate between fat necrosis and carcinoma. Mammography may not help either but ultrasound scan will often reveal characteristic features and a core biopsy or open biopsy is needed to confirm the diagnosis.

An irregular mass in the breast and relevant family history should always alert you to the possibility of a cancer. Diagnosis of a breast mass should be based on triple assessment:

- clinical examination
- radiological imaging
- biopsy (FNA, or core biopsy).

Mammography is typically employed in patients over 35, otherwise ultrasonography is used for diagnosis and can be combined with a guided biopsy. MRI is used for patients with breast implants.

41 c, c, a, a

In neonates the thymus is responsible for the development of T lymphocytes; in the adult it becomes a fat infiltrated remnant. Myasthenia gravis is an autoimmune disorder of peripheral nerves in which antibodies form against acetylcholine (ACh) postsynaptic receptors. Cholinergic nerve conduction to striated muscle is impaired by both mechanical blockage of the binding site by antibodies and by destruction of the postsynaptic receptor. Patients become symptomatic once the number of ACh receptors is reduced to approx. 30%. The earliest muscles involved are often those of the eyelids, those controlling eye movements and muscles controlling swallowing and speech. About 10% of cases are associated with a tumour of the thymus and most of the rest have thymic hyperplasia; the mechanism of the link revolves around T cell development, though is not fully understood presently. The thymus contains cells called Hassall's corpuscles.

Muscle contraction is dependent upon cumulative activation of the ACh receptors postsynaptically in the muscle; activation leads to a transport of calcium and sodium ions into the muscle and when levels of these ions are sufficient, contraction occurs. ACh, when released from the presynaptic cleft, is rapidly hydrolysed and inactivated. Thus, in myasthenia gravis where the number of postsynaptic receptors is reduced, the likelihood of a molecule of ACh reaching a receptor and activating it is vastly reduced. This causes the symptoms of rapid muscle fatigue.

In contrast, Lambert-Eaton syndrome is a presynaptic autoimmune disorder, in which auto-antibodies are directed against voltage-gated calcium channels. It is characterised by a muscle weakness, not usually affecting the muscles of the face, that improves as movement continues. In Lambert-Eaton, the presynaptic cleft is only able to release ACh at a low rate that may be insufficient to trigger the muscle to contract (below threshold). Therefore, repeated movement slowly builds up the triggering of ACh receptors postsynaptically, making movement progressively easier.

Therefore, treatment consists of a choline esterase inhibitor, e.g. pyridostigmine. This reduces the hydrolysation of ACh in the synapse, meaning that the likelihood of each molecule reaching a viable receptor is increased. Thyroidectomy is indicated if the tumour is invasive.

42 a, a, a, b

The adrenal glands are located superior and medial to the upper pole of each kidney. The two main components to the adrenals are the cortex and medulla. The cortex is divided into the:

- zona glomerulosa, the most superficial layer, secreting mineralo-corticoids, e.g. aldosterone
- zona fasciculata, the middle cortical layer, producing glucocorti-coids, e.g. cortisol
- zona reticularis, the deepest cortical layer, producing weak androgens.

All of these hormones are synthesised from cholesterol. The medulla produces catecholamines, epinephrine and norepinephrine in response to autonomic stimulation.

Conn's syndrome is characterised by the overproduction of aldos-terone (primary hyperaldosteronism), and results in sodium retention and potassium excretion. An aldosterone secreting adrenal adenoma (benign) is present, and is diagnosed on CT scan. Medical treatment involves the use of spironolactone, which competes with aldosterone on the distal tubule and the collecting duct. This is temporary until laparoscopic adrenalectomy can be performed.

43 a, a, a, a

When examining a thyroid several questions should be answered – is the swelling smooth or nodular? If it is nodular the number of nodules can be palpated. Any nodules palpated should also be assessed for size.

Diffusely swollen thyroids may be produced by iodine deficiency (iodine is required for producing thyroxine), Grave's disease, Hashimoto's thyroiditis and congenital abnormalities. Grave's disease is of clinical significance as the patient will be hyperthyroid – in this condition the body produces thyroid stimulating immunoglobulin which, as with TSH, stimulates the thyroid to produce more thyroxine.

Goitres with a single nodule can be due to a malignancy and this should be excluded; 10% of such nodules will be found to be malignant. Other benign lumps include colloid nodules and follicular nodules. If a nodule produces thyroxine without regard to TSH levels, it is known as an autonomous nodule. Investigation of such nodules involves ultrasound scanning and fine needle aspirate (FNA).

Multinodular goitres have more than one 'lump' causing swelling within the thyroid gland. These are normally euthyroid, however sometimes excessive T4 production results in hyperthyroidism (for example with a so-called toxic multinodular goitre). In most cases, the only symptoms are a painless swelling in the neck.

Treatment consists of radioactive iodine 131. Thyroidectomy is advised in patients with symptoms of tracheal compression. In younger patients it may be advisable to manage operatively, as there is a risk of haemorrhage into a thyroid cyst, leading to acute tracheal compression. The cosmetic appearance of a large neck mass may also prompt surgery.

Papillary carcinoma, approximately 60% of thyroid cancers, occurs in younger adults and adolescents. Typically subclinical, it occasionally may present due to a small asymptomatic nodule that has been felt by the patient.

Follicular adenoma is the second most prevalent (25%) and metastasises via the vascular system rather than lymphatics, having a worse prognosis. Medullary carcinoma (which may be associated with a phaeochromocytoma), together with thyroid lymphoma, make up a further 5% of prevalence each. Anaplastic carcinoma is the most aggressive, but rare, with early dissemination to regional lymphatics and bloodstream spreading to lungs, bone and brain.

44 c, c, a

The parathyroids (between 3–6 in number, most usually 4) produce parathyroid hormone (PTH), which regulates calcium and phosphate metabolism. PTH increases serum calcium by:

1 Stimulating bone resorption by indirectly stimulating osteoclasts.

2 Enhancing active reabsorption of calcium from the distal tubule and thick ascending limb in the kidney.

3 Enhancing intestinal absorption by increasing the production of activated vitamin D. PTH up-regulates the enzyme responsible for 1-α hydroxylation of 25-hydroxy vitamin D.

PTH also reduces the uptake of phosphate from the proximal tubule of the kidney, which means more phosphate is excreted through the urine.

Peribuccal tingling (surrounding the cheek) is an early sign of hypocalcaemia due to parathyroid removal. This can be treated with oral calcium and vitamin D supplements. Trousseau's sign is associated with hypocalcaemia. It is seen when a BP cuff is inflated to occlude the brachial artery and carpal spasm occurs. This is flexion at the wrist and metacarpophalangeal joints, extension of distal and proximal inter-phalangeal joints and adduction of the thumb.

45 b, a, e, b

Paraphimosis unfortunately can occur after catheterisation, resulting from retracting the foreskin which then acts as a constricting band preventing venous return. The swelling can then make it more difficult to replace the foreskin. Other causes include overretraction of the foreskin during erection. Relief is often achieved by using a local anaesthetic block and squeezing the glans until the foreskin can be reduced; if this fails a dorsal slit can be performed.

Phimosis is a narrowing of the preputial orifice. On micturition, the prepuce is seen to balloon and the stream is reduced to a dribble. Treatment is with circumcision. Balanitis is acute inflammation of the glans and foreskin usually due to coliform bacilli, staphylococci and streptococci. Diabetics are susceptible to *Candida* infections and this must be ruled out as treatment with antibiotics will not be effective. Balanitis can result in scarring and phimosis.

Carcinoma of the penis, while uncommon, may be inoperable if it spreads to the local lymphatics; treatment options would then be limited to palliation. The lesions are well differentiated squamous carcinomas and typically involve the inguinal lymph nodes bilaterally.

46 c, e, a, e

With a Glasgow Coma Score (GCS) of less than 8, the ability to maintain your own airway is severely compromised. A useful way of determining an approximate GCS quickly is with the AVPU system:

Alert
Voice (responsive to . . .)
Pain (responsive to . . .)
Unresponsive

If the patient is only responsive to pain then their GCS is approx. 8 and the airway will be threatened.

An immediate intervention would be the placement of a Guedel airway if you are not adequately trained in the other methods listed. A nasopharyngeal airway is often tolerated better by semiconscious patients, however in this case, with a history of head trauma, a Guedel would be the more appropriate option. High flow oxygen should be administered in addition.

The diagnosis is likely to be a subdural haematoma, with the mechanism described and no lucid interval. In light of the INR of 8, prothrombin complex, together with vitamin K, is now the immediate treatment administered; it reverses the effects of warfarin more rapidly than FFP and requires less volume to be administered.

47 b, e, a, a, b

While a plain kidneys, ureters and bladder (KUB) radiograph will demonstrate the presence of ureteric calculi in 90% of cases, a CT KUB is more sensitive, and is replacing intravenous urograms (IVU) at many centres as the investigation of choice. The added benefit is that other pathology can also be sought. MAG3 renography can demonstrate renal impairment as well as obstruction.

Pethidine is said to be the analgesic of choice for both ureteric and biliary colic as it does not cause sphincter spasm, thereby worsening the symptoms, as can happen with morphine. Diclofenac may also be considered if not contraindicated. If the stone is not passed then extracorporeal shockwave lithotripsy is the first line treatment, the other options listed can be used if this is unsuccessful.

Proteus infection, which causes the urine to become more alkaline due to urease enzyme, predisposes to calcium phosphate crystals.

48 c, d, b, a

Haematuria while on anticoagulation is still more commonly due to urinary tract pathology that the anticoagulation has made symptomatic. All of the investigations listed are used to find a cause for haematuria. IVU is useful for looking for an obstruction and urine MCS will identify an infective cause. USS is able to demonstrate parenchymal tumours, and lesions in the collecting system. However flexible cystoscopy with local anaesthetic is the most valuable investigation as a biopsy of any lesion found may be taken at the same time for definitive diagnosis.

Transitional cell carcinoma is responsible for 90% of primary malignant bladder cancers. Risk factors include smoking and β-naphthalene (once used in the rubber and plastics industry). Surgical treatment is via transurethral resection depending on the stage. For high-grade tumours intravesical chemotherapy may be used postoperatively to prevent recurrence.

49 d, a, b

Prostate enlargement has been reported as being common from the age of 45 but is symptomatic in 70% by the age of 70. The enlargement can lead to extrinsic compression of the urethra, leading to outflow obstruction. As a result this can cause:

- trabeculation of the bladder
- bladder diverticula
- bladder stones
- urinary tract infection.

Medical therapy for moderately or severely symptomatic patients includes selective α-1 adrenergic antagonists that cause relaxation of smooth muscle at the bladder neck, an example being tamsulosin. 5α-reductase inhibitors prevent testosterone being converted to dihydrotestosterone, which is believed to be responsible for the increase in prostate growth.

If this fails then a transurethral resection of the prostate (TURP) is indicated. This is not without complications, including haemorrhage, infection and retrograde ejaculation. TURP syndrome is the result of the absorption of large volumes of irrigating fluid used during the procedure; this can lead to a profound hyponatraemia and consequent cerebral oedema.

50 b, b, d, e

Isografts are a subset of allografts which involve donation to a genetically identical recipient, e.g. a monozygotic twin. Allografts refer to transplants between members of the same species while autografts involve site to site transplantation from the same person, e.g. skin, or vein grafts. Xenografts are between different species, e.g. porcine heart valves.

The position of the organ graft is described by the terms orthotopic and heterotopic. An orthotopic graft is placed in an anatomically normal position, for example in heart transplantation. A heterotopic graft is implanted in a non-anatomical position; kidney transplantation is achieved by placing the donor kidney in the iliac fossa thus making this procedure a heterotopic graft.

There are several exclusion criteria in place to ensure the relative safety of the recipient and prevent the transfer of disease from the donor, for example malignancy. However, a low-grade primary brain tumour is not considered to be a contraindication to transplant. Some centres are increasingly performing transplants without ABO or HLA compatibility between recipient and donor, though most programmes attempt a compatible cross match.

Prognosis following renal transplant is very good, with 1-year survival at approximately 95% (or greater for allografts) and a 5-year survival between 70 and 80%, again with better figures for allografts.

51 c, b, a, b

Haemosiderin deposition, lipodermatosclerosis, varicose eczema and ulceration are all common skin changes associated with varicose veins. Haemosiderin deposition is caused by loss of red blood cells into the tissues and consequent release of haemoglobin. Lipodermatosclerosis is the term given to skin and subcutaneous tissue changes caused by chronic venous hypertension – this is a progressive sclerosis of both skin and subcutaneous fat by fibrin deposition, tissue death and scarring.

One of the best surgical treatments for varicose veins is high tie and vein stripping. However if there is deep vein insufficiency and one removes the superficial veins, symptoms will worsen. For this reason, ultrasound scanning is performed before surgery. It should be noted that mixed disease ulcers (i.e. those of both an arterial and venous origin) require ABPI assessment before four-layer compression stockings are used to avoid an iatrogenic reduction in arterial supply to an ischaemic limb.

The most common site of venous incompetence is at the saphenofemoral junction. Other common sites are at the junction of the short saphenous popliteal junction and also the perforator veins between the superficial and deep system.

52 d, d, a, b

Poliovirus is an RNA virus that is transmitted through the faecal-oral route or by ingestion of contaminated water. After a period of viraemia, the virus becomes neurotropic and causes destruction of the anterior horn cells. This destruction leads to development of flaccid paralysis.

Two types of vaccine are routinely used in the prevention of poliomyelitis; inactivated poliovirus and oral attenuated poliovirus vaccine.

The knee abnormality is genu varus; genu recurvatum and is more prevalent in patients with connective tissue disorders. Trendelenburg's test is useful in identifying abductor weakness of the hip, resulting in the dipping of the pelvis on the unaffected side.

53 a, b, b, c

This is a likely venous ulcer; the dilated superficial veins are probably varicose and there is a classic gaiter/medial malleolus distribution. A Marjolin's ulcer is a squamous cell carcinoma that occurs in chronically inflamed or scarred skin; classically it is described as having 'heaped' edges. Curling's ulcers typically occur after severe burns, whereas a Cushing's ulcer is a gastric ulcer produced by elevated intracranial pressure, thought to be due to stimulation of the vagal nuclei causing increased secretion of gastric acid. Arterial ulcers are typically accompanied by other symptoms and signs of arterial insufficiency in the peripheries, for example weak or absent peripheral pulses.

Compression stockings are the treatment of choice after arterial insufficiency has been ruled out; this could be achieved by obtaining an ABPI or carrying out a duplex ultrasound.

Compression stockings are a four-layer system applied by a specialist nurse, consisting of:

1 A non-adherent dressing to protect the ulcer.
2 Wool to cushion the dressing and protect the vulnerable surrounding skin.
3 Graduated compression bandages – the functional component of the dressing which encourages venous return. It runs from foot to thigh.
4 Tubular bandages – an elastic bandage which merely keeps the whole dressing in place and stops the compression bandage from unravelling.

54 a, c, b, a

Dry gangrene is likely and is primarily caused as a result of ischaemia. The distinct black colour is due to the release of haemoglobin from the red cells which is subsequently metabolised; bacteria with hydrogen sulphide produce black iron sulphide that remains in the tissue.

Gangrene, if caught early enough can be reversed if revascularisation is achieved. If the gangrene is uncomplicated, i.e. it is not wet or the patient is not compromised, then auto-amputation is the most appropriate management.

Diabetes is a microvascular disease; this can lead to ischaemic disease in the peripheries due to a diseased capillary system. Pedal pulses may be palpable as the macrovascular circulation (i.e. arteries and arterioles) will remain patent.

Often the ankle brachial pressure index will be > 1 owing to the increased opening pressure required for the diseased and calcified vessels. If the compressible pressure of the pulse is < 50 mmHg this indicates critical ischaemia.

55 b, a, c, b

This mass is above the umbilicus which lies at approximately L4. L4 is commonly referred to as the point at which the aorta bifurcates to form the common iliac vessels. Therefore, this pulsatile, expansile mass is an abdominal aortic aneurysm until proven otherwise. Ultrasonography is a good modality for initial diagnosis and screening whereas computerised tomography (CT) scanning can delineate the precise location, vessel involvement and size.

The UK small aneurysm trial indicated that the risk of aneurysmal rupture exceeded the risk of elective open aneurysm repair when the aneurysm had a diameter > 5.5 cm. Endoscopic vascular repair can be considered if a patient's aneurysm is 1 cm infrarenal and has a clear zone of 1.4 cm at the distal end.

Aortic aneurysms represent a degenerative process often attributed to atherosclerosis. Other causes include Marfan's syndrome, Ehlers-Danlos syndrome, syphilis and mycotic aneurysms.

56 a, b, b, a

This patient has an arteriovenous fistula between the radial artery and the cephalic vein, created surgically for ease of vascular access in patients with renal failure requiring dialysis or filtration. There are various methods and sites of creating a fistula, some of the most common being autogenous (using a vein graft) or using synthetic straight grafts. Other sites include the brachial artery and the cephalic vein, with distal sites considered first. Examination would show a dilated pulsatile, expansile mass in the non-dominant arm. Auscultation of the mass would reveal a machinery murmur.

Postoperative complications include nerve injury, particularly the radial and median nerves. If the hand becomes swollen without pain this may indicate a venous thrombosis. This may be due to poor flow, disruption of the course of the vessels, or to venous compression by a haematoma.

Steal phenomenon may occur due to flow following the path of least resistance down the venous system, causing the distal portion to become inadequately perfused. This leads to ischaemia-like symptoms, with a painful hand.

57 d, e, a, e

This is a popliteal artery aneurysm as it is a pulsatile, expansile mass sited in the popliteal fossa. Popliteal aneurysms are typically confirmed by ultrasound scan and account for 80% of all peripheral aneurysms. Fifty per cent are bilateral and 50% are asymptomatic. The symptomatic aneurysms present due to compression or rupture of adjacent structures. Treatment if symptomatic is by proximal and distal ligation, with revascularisation of the leg achieved via a femoropopliteal bypass. Asymptomatic aneurysms are not surgically treated until the diameter is greater than 2 cm, or they become symptomatic.

A Baker's cyst is a fluctuant swelling in the popliteal fossa. It is a synovial sac bulging from the back of the joint. It is not pulsatile. If the cyst leaks then this may cause pain and swelling that is similar to that of a DVT. The two can be differentiated by ultrasound scan.

58 b, c, a, c

Dercum's disease, otherwise known as adiposis dolorosa, is a condition characterised by multiple lipomas. The lipomas are associated with pressure to the nerves, resulting in pain. The condition is different to familial multiple lipomas, which is an autosomal dominant condition characterised by multiple asymptomatic lipomas. Observation is the most appropriate management, with analgesia and surgical excision of troublesome lesions.

Leser-Trelat syndrome is the rapid eruption of multiple seborrheic keratoses in the presence of intra-abdominal malignancy. Sister Joseph's nodule is found in the umbilicus and indicates an underlying malignancy; it is due to secondary spread, either from the liver along the falciform ligament or from the pelvic organs along the various ligamentous attachments to the umbilicus.

Klippel-Trenaunay syndrome consists of a triad of symptoms:

- varicose veins
- port-wine stain
- soft issue hypertrophy.

This normally affects a single extremity, usually the leg, followed by the arms. Treatment is usually conservative and reserved for symptomatic episodes; compression garments, analgesia and antibiotics are typically used if required. Debulking procedures are limited as they may damage venous and lymphatic structures.

59 a, c, a, b

This elderly patient is likely to have a ruptured proximal biceps tendon. Upon active elbow flexion against resistance, the belly of the biceps will contract to form a prominent lump. This rupture is normally limited to the long head of biceps due to degeneration; it does not require surgical intervention. Rupture of the distal tendon, associated with trauma, does require surgical intervention to restore function.

A ruptured Achilles tendon can be assessed by Simmond's test, in which the patient is asked to kneel on the chair, facing away from the examiner, and the calf squeezed. If the tendon is ruptured the foot will not plantar flex.

While treatment for tendon rupture can be conservative, younger, physically active patients can benefit from prompt surgical intervention.

60 b, a, d, e

Any lesion that has brought a patient to clinic should be taken seriously. The red flags should further that suspicion and prompt rapid excision and histological analysis. The red flags are:

A – asymmetry
B – border (irregularity) and bleeding
C – colour (variegated)
D – diameter (> 6 mm or increasing in size)

There are four common types of melanoma:

1   Superficial spreading – this is the most common type and can occur on any part of the body but is more prevalent on the sun exposed areas and in fairer skin.

2   Nodular melanoma – often protrudes with a smooth surface; it may become ulcerated or bleed.

3   Lentigo maligna melanoma – arises from a Hutchinson's lentigo.

4   Acral lentigious melanoma – the commonest type in black patients; an irregular expanding area of brown or black pigmentation on the palm, sole or beneath the nail.

Examination must be thorough: top to toe including all lymph nodes. If no lymph nodes are detected surgical excision must be performed and histology sent and acted upon. If lymph nodes are found and are positive on biopsy, surgical clearance +/- chemotherapy or radiotherapy may be necessary.

61 c, a, b, d

Raynaud's phenomenon refers to symptoms that occur secondary to other causes, whereas Raynaud's disease, often called primary Raynaud's, is diagnosed if no other cause can be found. Reynaud's disease is more prevalent in young girls. Both conditions have the characteristic white, blue and crimson skin colour changes when the extremities are exposed to cold temperatures. This is painful and in severe form can be associated with digital ulcers.

Raynaud's phenomenon can be attributed to a variety of causes, including occupational exposure to vibrating tools, medications such as the oral contraceptive pill, and cigarette smoking. Raynaud's can form part of the CREST syndrome (calcinosis, Raynaud's, oesophageal dysmotility, sclerodactyly and telangiectasia).

Treatment is often conservative, with the use of heated gloves and lifestyle changes, including smoking cessation. Medical management includes nifedipine and prostacyclins if that fails. Surgical intervention using sympathectomy may be used in severe non-responsive cases.

62 a, b, b, c

Hyperhidrosis as a condition is characterised by increased perspiration and can be generalised or localised. The hands, feet and axilla are most commonly affected. Medical treatment involves the use initially of aluminium hydroxide. If this fails, Botox injections can be used. If medical treatment fails, sympathectomy can be used but as with all surgical procedures there are risks, e.g. Horner's syndrome. Hyperhidrosis erythematous traumatica is a rare occupational form of the condition in which sweating occurs in skin which is in contact with vibrating tools.

Hidradenitis suppurativa is an infection of the apocrine glands often in the axilla and groin. The condition is chronic, with initial management centred around incision and drainage of the abscess with possible definitive treatment involving radical excision and skin grafting in severe cases. Long-term metronidazole may be used to control flare ups.

Frey's syndrome can occur following parotid surgery. The auriculotemporal branch of the mandibular nerve carries sympathetic fibres to the sweat glands of the scalp and parasympathetic fibres to the parotid gland. Severance and inappropriate regeneration can result in 'gustatory sweating', or sweating in the anticipation of eating, instead of the normal salivatory response.

63 c, d

Incisional hernias develop as a late complication in about 10% of all abdominal surgery. Usually the incisional hernia presents as a 'bulge' in the abdominal wall near a previous incision. The condition is often asymptomatic but, as with all forms of hernia, can become strangulated if the neck is narrow, leading to the contents becoming ischaemic. Once developed the hernia tends to enlarge gradually and can impact on the patient's daily life, such as making dressing difficult.

This patient gives a history of intermittent incarceration and obstruction. This should therefore be repaired electively with laparoscopic surgery becoming a favoured option; a large mesh is placed over the defect rather than the defect being closed.

64 d, b, e, c

A hydrocele is an abnormal quantity of serous fluid within the tunica vaginalis. The fluid is commonly around the testis, as it collects in the process vaginalis which means the testicle cannot be palpated separately. The cause is commonly primary, which is a gradual accumulation of fluid seen in children or the elderly. Secondary hydroceles appear rapidly and are associated with trauma, epididymo-orchitis and tumour, among others.

A varicocele consists of dilated pampiniform plexus veins. Patients who are symptomatic often describe a dragging or aching sensation. The sudden appearance of a varicocele should raise the suspicion of retroperitoneal disease.

Testicular cancer has a peak at 25–35 years of age and commonly presents as a painless mass in the scrotum. It is worth noting that lymphatic spread is to the para-aortic lymph nodes rather than the inguinal nodes, which drain the scrotal skin. The most appropriate tumour markers are α-fetoprotein (AFP) and human chorionic gonadotropin (HCG). Epididymal cysts are a fluid-filled swelling of a benign nature containing opaque fluid with spermatozoa. They are usually asymptomatic but may develop pain.

65 b, d, d

This patient has a colostomy. The single most important clue is that the stoma is not spouted; ileostomies are spouted, whereas colostomies are flat. Other important clues are the site, with ileostomies typically placed on the right iliac fossa and colostomies on the left. The content of the appliance is also key; liquid green effluent is likely to be small bowel content; formed stool indicates colostomy; urine a urostomy.

There are many complications associated with a stoma; this patient is suffering from a parastomal hernia. Others include ischaemia, stenosis prolapse, bypassing the proximal loop and entering the distal loop.

Parastomal hernias may contain bowel at risk of obstruction and/or strangulation. As this patient is stable, an elective repair, which normally takes the form of resiting the stoma, may be taken. This may include the placement of a mesh to try and reduce the risk of recurrence.

66 b, a, a

The diagnosis is likely primary osteoarthritis, i.e. when no other underlying cause can be identified. Other causes of osteoarthritis of the hip are congenital subluxation, Perthes' disease or acetabular deformities in young patients. In older patients it may be secondary to rheumatoid arthritis, avascular necrosis or Paget's disease.

Apparent shortening (as in this case) is measured with the patient supine, both anterior superior iliac spines (ASIS) parallel. The distance measured is the distance from the umbilicus to the medial malleolus. Apparent shortening is caused by fixed flexion or adduction deformity. True shortening is caused by the actual affected limb being physically shorter than the other. Measurement is made from the ASIS to the medial malleolus. The affected part of the lower limb can be further identified by flexing the knee and observing any discrepancy.

Thomas's test is used to demonstrate fixed flexion of the pelvis. The examiner's hand is placed under the lumbar spine and the hip flexed until the lumbar curve is felt against the hand. In a normal hip, no further movement will be seen. In the affected hip, there will be movement off the couch.

67 a, c, b, d

Perthes' test involves placing a tourniquet around the leg that occludes the superficial venous system; any venous return is then drained by the deep venous system only, as it would if the patient had surgical disconnection of the saphenofemoral junction. Venous return is then encouraged by asking the patient to stand up and down on their toes. If the deep system is not patent or the valves are incompetent then there will be engorgement of the limb, and the patient will experience a bursting pain as the veins fill. This test illustrates why it is important to check the patency of the deep system before carrying out varicose vein surgery.

The level of valve incompetence can be determined by the emptying of the venous system by elevating the affected leg, the placement of a tourniquet, and then asking the patient to stand. If this fails to control the superficial veins, the process is repeated and the tourniquet placed at a different level.

Trendelenburg's test involves emptying the venous system as above, then placement of pressure over the saphenofemoral junction. This is difficult to perform in practice and is seldom performed. Buerger's test demonstrates arterial insufficiency and when the leg becomes reperfused on resting the leg over the edge of the couch, reactive hyperaemia is observed.

68 b, e, b, b

In an acute flare-up of rheumatoid arthritis, there is often an effusion present and thickened synovium. The joint is usually tender. Genu recurvatum is often associated with connective tissue disorders, e.g. Ehlers-Danlos syndrome, which is seen as hyperextension of the knee upon standing.

Osgood-Schlatter occurs in the 10–16 age group, presenting as recurrent pain over the tibial tuberosity. The condition is thought to be due to multiple subacute avulsion fractures. This usually resolves once the epiphyseal growth plates have fused. Treatment should be conservative and initially restricted to analgesia.

Osteochondritis dissecans, a form of osteochondrosis, is a painful joint condition in which a fragment of cartilage becomes loose within the joint (so-called joint mice) leading to inflammation and pain.

69 b, a, b, a

Osteoarthritis of the hands is associated with bony swellings around the distal interphalangeal joints; these are known as Heberden's nodes. Nodes at the proximal interphalangeal joints are Bouchard's nodes. Rheumatoid nodules are often seen around the elbows. Other extra-articular features can be seen in the eyes, e.g. episcleritis; chest signs, e.g. fibrosing alveolitis; cardiac signs, e.g. pericarditis; abdominal signs, e.g. splenomegaly in Felty's syndrome.

There are three deformities of the digits. Boutonniere deformity is hyperflexion of the proximal interphalangeal joints with fixed extension of the metacarpophalangeal and distal interphalangeal joints. Swan neck is hyperextension of the proximal interphalangeal joint. 'Z thumb' deformity is hyperextension of the metacarpophalangeal joint.

70 a, a, e

Dupuytren's contracture is a painless nodular thickening and contracture of the palmar aponeurosis, particularly on the ulnar side, extending distally to involve the little and ring fingers. This causes a fixed flexion deformity at the metacarpophalangeal joints. This deformity has been linked to a ZF9 gene mutation; ZF9 maps to chromosome 10P, near the telomere. Other causes that have been proposed include alcoholic liver disease, trauma, manual labour, diabetes and drugs.

Other features are Garrod's pads, which are knuckle pads. Other associated aponeurotic thickening conditions are Peyronie's disease of the penis and Ledderhose's disease of the plantar aponeurosis.

Functional deficit is assessed by Houston's test, which involves placing the hand palm down on a table, thus measuring the degree of functional impairment. Combined with patient wishes, this can be used to determine the need for surgical management.

71 d, b, c, a

The long thoracic nerve supplies serratus anterior, which prevents winging of the scapula. This can be demonstrated by asking the patient to place their hands against a wall and the prominent scapula in question is observed.

Asking the patient to point their thumb at the ceiling with their hand on a flat surface tests for the median nerve and, in particular, the abductor pollicis brevis. Other specific muscles in the hand supplied by the median nerve are the lateral two lumbricals, opens pollicis and flexor pollicis brevis.

Froment's test is for adductor pollicis which is supplied by the ulnar nerve. The patient is asked to hold a sheet of paper between their thumb and index finger, with their thumb on top. The examiner then copies this and pulls the paper away. If there is a lesion of the adductor pollicis the thumb will flex at the interphalangeal joint, using the thumb flexors to compensate.

Sensory testing of the radial nerve is best demonstrated over the first web space, which is between the thumb and the index finger.

72 b, a, e, c

In the hand, the ulnar nerve is primarily responsible for sensation of the little finger, the ulnar half of the ring finger and the ulnar border of the hand. It has two branches in the hand: the deep and superficial branches. The deep branch innervates the hypothenar muscles (together providing movement of the little finger), adductor pollicis (providing adduction of the thumb), the third and fourth lumbricals (which maintain extension of the little and ring fingers) and the dorsal and palmar interossei (which abduct and adduct the fingers respectively).

The patient in this case has point tenderness over the little finger metacarpal; the ideal view of the metacarpal is achieved with an AP and oblique radiograph of the right hand – finger views will be inadequately centred and may not show the whole metacarpal. A lateral view will not be useful due to the overlap of the other metacarpals.

Angulation of a neck of metacarpal fracture that is less than 15° may be treated conservatively with an ulnar gutter splint, with mobilisation at the 2-week point. A fracture clinic appointment should be booked for this time, to reassess the fracture and ensure acceptable union is taking place. Any angulation of greater than 15° should be reduced.

The fracture described is often called a boxer's fracture in view of the fact that it is normally sustained by the patient striking a solid object with his or her fist, for example a wall or another individual's skull. Patients with this injury may have poor recall of events leading up to the injury, often due to accompanying alcohol intake, or may deliberately withhold information making them poor historians.

73 b, d, a, a

The usual order of ossification in the paediatric elbow can be recalled by use of the mnemonic CRITOL:

- Capitellum
- Radial head
- Internal (medial epicondyle)
- Trochlea
- Olecranon
- Lateral epicondyle

The majority (95%) of supracondylar fractures are extension-type fractures and are graded using the Gartland system of classification. This system recognises three grades of fracture: grade I is undisplaced, grade II is displaced though with an intact posterior cortex, and grade III is displaced with no cortical contact.

While distal radial fractures can occur concomitantly with supracondylar fractures in 5–6% of cases, the most important assessment is the distal limb neurovascular status. Median nerve injuries are the most common, followed by radial and then ulnar lesions. Vascular compromise can also occur and may depend upon the position of the limb until definitive reduction can take place.

This patient has a completely displaced supracondylar fracture, i.e. a Gartland grade III. The definitive management would be to proceed to an MUA and internal fixation with K-wires. If reduction via this method is not possible, or there is neurovascular compromise, it may become necessary to convert to an open reduction.

74 a, d, d, c, a

This scenario, although not common, does occur. Diverticular abscess is a common general surgical problem, for which conservative management with antibiotics is often trialled, providing certain criteria are met. These patients can become septic and subsequently develop circulatory collapse secondary to septic shock.

Early aggressive fluid challenge is important and should be guided by the BP, pulse rate and end organ perfusion, such as cerebration (confusion, GCS) and kidney perfusion (a urine output of greater than 0.5 mL/kg/hr). The key to managing this patient is not to be satisfied by 30 mL/hr but to act early to prevent disaster.

Simple measures such as fluid challenge and head down can all help bring the BP up, but ultimately the only way to treat this patient will be to remove the source of infection, either by percutaneous drainage or a Hartmann's procedure and abdominal washout. However, this patient has continued to deteriorate and, with a GCS of less than 8, her airway will now be compromised and an adjunct such as a Guedel airway should be placed and a cardiac arrest call should be made.

The rhythm is ventricular fibrillation and the algorithm for treatment is set out by the Resuscitation Council as per the Advanced Life Support Algorithm for shockable rhythms. While the diagnosis is being made, compressions and ventilation via bag valve mask should be made at a ratio of 30 compressions to 2 breaths. Once leads are on and a shockable rhythm is diagnosed a shock of 150 J biphasic should be delivered. After the second cycle and before the third shock, 1 mg adrenaline IV should be given. During this time the reversible causes should be addressed; in this case the most likely cause is hypovolaemia secondary to systemic inflammatory response syndrome.

75 a, b, d

It is often the case that you will be unable to obtain a complete past medical and surgical history from patients when they attend acutely to the Emergency Department, as it is in this question.

All we know about this gentleman is that he is hypothermic, tachycardic, hypotensive and hypoxic. He is likely a long-term smoker as evidenced by the tar staining of his fingers. Of all his unstable observations the value that is most urgent to address is his hypoxia (as per the ABCDE approach). We know he is a smoker and he may or may not have respiratory disease. Regardless, the correct treatment is high-flow oxygen, delivered at 15 litres per minute via a non-rebreather bag and mask. This delivers oxygen at approximately 75–85%.

The patient's ABG demonstrates an acidosis (low pH, < 7.35) and a raised carbon dioxide level (> 6.0). His oxygen is in the normal range, though would be hypoxic for the amount of oxygen he is receiving. The acidosis has been caused by the high carbon dioxide and is hence respiratory in nature. He has a high bicarbonate, suggesting that his kidneys have made some attempt at compensating for the acidosis. This would suggest that the current acute process has been going on for at least 48 hours, since it will take that amount of time for renal bicarbonate excretion rates to adjust.

With the evidence we have managed to gather, the most likely diagnosis is one of an infective exacerbation of chronic obstructive airways disease; hypothermia, tachycardia and hypotension can be explained by sepsis and respiratory features and blood gas by carbon dioxide retention of COPD. He will ultimately require surgery for the fractured neck of femur, but should first be stabilised by the use of nebulisers, intravenous antibiotics, oxygen titration and repeat ABG monitoring and, if necessary, BiPAP.

Index

Note: questions and answers are given in the following format Q/A

T - #0563 - 101024 - C0 - 234/156/10 - PB - 9781846192678 - Gloss Lamination